Ethics in Healthcare

Ethics in Healthcare

A Philosophical Introduction

Ezio Di Nucci

ROWMAN &
LITTLEFIELD
INTERNATIONAL
London • New York

Executive Editor: Isobel Cowper-Coles
Associate Editor: Natalie Bolderston

Credits and acknowledgments for material borrowed from other sources, and reproduced with permission, appear on the appropriate page within the text.

Published by Rowman & Littlefield International, Ltd.
Unit A, Whitacre Mews, 26-34 Stannary Street, London SE11 4AB
www.rowmaninternational.com

Rowman & Littlefield International, Ltd., is an affiliate of
Rowman & Littlefield
4501 Forbes Boulevard, Suite 200, Lanham, Maryland 20706, USA
With additional offices in Boulder, New York, Toronto (Canada), and Plymouth (UK)
www.rowman.com

British Library Cataloguing in Publication Data

A catalogue record for this book is available from the British Library

ISBN: HB 978-1-78660-869-7
PB 978-1-78660-870-3

Library of Congress Cataloging-in-Publication Data

Names: Di Nucci, Ezio, author.
Title: Ethics in healthcare : a philosophical introduction / Ezio Di Nucci.
Description: London ; New York : Rowman & Littlefield International, Ltd., [2018] | Includes bibliographical references and index.
Identifiers: LCCN 2018018383 (print) | LCCN 2018022015 (ebook) | ISBN 9781786608710 (Electronic) | ISBN 9781786608697 (HB : alk. paper) | ISBN 9781786608703 (PB : alk. paper)
Subjects: LCSH: Medical ethics. | Clinical medicine—Decision making.
Classification: LCC R725 (ebook) | LCC R725 .D5 2018 (print) | DDC 174.2—dc23 LC record available at https://lccn.loc.gov/2018018383

∞ ™ The paper used in this publication meets the minimum requirements of American National Standard for Information Sciences—Permanence of Paper for Printed Library Materials, ANSI/NISO Z39.48–1992.
Printed in the United States of America

a Caterina, Eleonore, Franz e Ursula

Contents

Acknowledgements

I must first of all thank my students at the University of Copenhagen, who have contributed in many (explicit and implicit) ways to this book, way beyond just motivating me to write it in the first place. This book is therefore not only for them but also very much by them. I also ought to thank past and present members of the SUND philosophy group here at the University of Copenhagen; a lot of the material here is the result of our continuing collaboration in teaching ethics and philosophy to healthcare students: Morten Hillgaard Bülow, Annamaria Carusi, Martin Ejsing Christensen, Jan Kyrre Berg Friis, Sara Green, Finn Guldmann, Henrik Harksen, Rasmus Thybo Jensen, Jeanette Bresson Ladegaard Knox, Christopher Jamil de Montgomery, Lars Poulsen, Peter Rossel, Elise Utke Schiøler, Anders Tversted Silber, and Peter Laurs Sørensen—special thanks go to Rasmus for his revisions and to Jeanette for her daily support! Thanks also to all my wonderful colleagues at the Department of Public Health, especially Henriette Langstrup and Klaus Høyer. Also from my department, thanks to Anna Vera Jørring Pallesen for help with the index. Thanks to everyone at Rowman and Littlefield, especially Natalie Bolderston and Isobel Cowper-Coles and the three anonymous reviewers. Also thanks to all those who have contributed to the Danish edition of this book (*Ethics4Medics: En guide til sundhedsfagene*): especially Laura Norn Hammen and Liva Skogemann. There are also a large number of philosophers around the world to which I owe a debt of gratitude, both intellectual and often also personal; but since I don't know where to start, let's just say I don't like name-dropping. And finally thanks to Ursula, obviously.

List of Case Studies

Introduction

What is ethics? And why should healthcare students and professionals care about it? This book tries to answer these questions in a way which is both accessible and, hopefully, interesting to people with no previous training in philosophy. I am not going to summarize my answer in this short introduction: I am afraid you will have to actually read the book, no shortcuts. But I will say that it is more than a little bit embarrassing for a philosopher to want to talk (let alone teach) ethics to healthcare students and professionals. I am familiar with this feeling because it comes back to me at the beginning of every new semester when I welcome a new cohort of aspiring doctors at the University of Copenhagen. It is my students—not I—who have chosen a career dedicated to helping others and that will go on—I am sure—to do a lot of good. This makes my job much easier, because I am preaching to the converted, so to speak.

Still, ethical questions and dilemmas do not exhaust all the different philosophical problems crucial to healthcare, as we will see in this book. And, more importantly, wanting to do good is a very good start but it provides very little in terms of answers to ethical questions: What constitutes doing good in a particular situation? And according to which overall principles? Must you always respect your patients' wishes, for example? What about those times when (you think) you know better? What about hard cases such as euthanasia and assisted suicide? Healthcare professionals are faced with difficult decisions every day, sometimes impossible ones; if their training is to provide any guidance and support in navigating such situations, then it must also include some ethics and philosophy—it is to that part of medical education that this book aspires to make a contribution.

I don't want to say much more in this introduction, but I would like to clarify what kind of book you can expect: this is not an introduction to bioethics or medical ethics. There are plenty of those around, starting from the modern classic *Principles of Biomedical Ethics* by Tom L. Beauchamp and James F. Childress.[1] My book is both much broader and much less detailed than an introduction to medical ethics ever ought to be: it rather aims to provide a guide for healthcare students and healthcare professionals to the way in which ethics and philosophy can be important to them and their professions—be that doctors, nurses, researchers, or other healthcare workers. I am sure that more than once throughout the book my seven readers will have to wonder about the relevance of some of the questions I address or distinctions I make: but the fundamental character of some of the material in this book is just a reflection of the difficult questions that readers will have to deal with in their professional lives.

Finally, a few words on the structure of the book: it contains eight chapters, reflecting the eight two-hour lectures that make up my *Ethics and Philosophy of Medicine* course, which I have been delivering to medical students at the University of Copenhagen since 2015. Teaching students is the greatest pleasure and honour of my job; in this case it also happens to have been an invaluable resource in writing this little book.

Note

1. Tom L. Beauchamp and James F. Childress, *Principles of Biomedical Ethics*. Seventh edition (Oxford University Press, 2012).

CHAPTER ONE

Mind and World

What's the Point of Philosophy Anyway?

You may be wondering why on earth healthcare professionals should bother with ethics and philosophy. What is the point of it? Those are actually two separate questions: what's the point of philosophy and ethics in general, and what is the point of them when it comes to the healthcare context? Both are, I think, legitimate questions—so I will start by trying to provide an answer; and this will also end up giving an introduction to the subject matter of this book.

There are, I think, at least two ways of showing the importance of philosophy and philosophical questions even for those who work (or will go on to work) within healthcare; and, more in general, for those with practical or applied tasks and jobs—otherwise known as 'the real world' (as philosophers like to call, well, everything else really).

I. The first point is that empirical questions (and answers) do not exhaust all the questions worth asking (whether they may still exhaust all the answers though, at least all the meaningful ones anyway, is a more difficult issue).
II. Secondly, a lot of your work within healthcare will consist in decision making and problem solving, and many of the tools and skills that are necessary for effective decision making and problem solving are the tools of reason—they are, namely, philosophical tools and skills.

This second point is exacerbated by technological progress and automation, which at the same time reduce the manual tasks for which professionals (as in, *human* professionals) are required while also increasing the complexity of the decisions that human professionals have to make and the problems that they have to solve. Technological development may offer exciting new therapeutic possibilities and certainly provides overall for better healthcare, but that does not at the same time necessarily mean that it makes the working lives of healthcare professionals easier; the very opposite may actually be the case.

Each of the above two points is enough to independently show the importance of philosophy as a discipline and of philosophical questions in particular; both generally speaking and specifically for doctors and healthcare professionals. But while I will not elaborate on the second issue here, this chapter will concern itself with the first point.

Empirical Questions Are Not All the Questions Worth Asking

It is easy to show that many questions, many important questions, are not empirical questions and that the fact that they cannot be solved empirically is no reason not to ask and try to answer these questions—that, you may say, is what philosophy is for.

Try to think of what matters most to you and you will see that some if not many of the things we hold most dear are not empirical: am I going to die? Yes, you are. This is indeed pretty high on anybody's list while being, admittedly, an empirical issue—both science and experience show us the inevitability of death. Does god exist? It very likely does not, but already here it is not obvious that this question can be settled empirically. Or think about questions such as whether to have children or what career to choose: many of the great practical questions in our lives are not easily settled empirically. Not to mention ethical dilemmas: Why should one do the right thing? What's in it for me? Again, if there is an answer, it does not look to be a simple question of fact.

More philosophically, 'Why is there something rather than nothing?' is a question that most people will have posed themselves at some point during their lives and it is, according to some (notably Martin Heidegger), *the* most fundamental question; but it is hardly a question that we can answer empirically through scientific method or experiments.

In somewhat similar terms we could think of questions about the finite or infinite nature of time and space; think of those deep questions from our childhood about what's beyond the end of the universe or what was before the beginning of it.

The same goes for epistemological questions about whether we can ever know the external world or be sure that it—or anything really—does actually exist: recall Rene Descartes' *cogito ergo sum*, according to which the only thing that we cannot doubt is our own existence as thinking beings; as minds, that is, rather than bodies. So we can't even be sure of the existence of our own body, according to Descartes, let alone the rest of the universe.

But we don't even need to go to these great depths of fundamentality to encounter nonempirical questions: if you were asked to point your index finger at your mind, in which direction would you point? You may plausibly answer that you would point towards your head for the simple reason that the mind is either identical with the brain, or anyway somewhat dependent on or connected to the brain (or at least more generally to our body anyway). These are plausible answers that are the object of much debate within philosophy; but again here the point is not what the correct answer is but what kind of question we are asking and what kinds of answers would be legitimate or appropriate ones in the first place—and the suggestion we are looking at is that what the mind is and what its relation to the brain consists of are not purely empirical questions that can be settled through scientific method alone.[1]

CASE STUDY 1: The Nervous Patient

More specifically to the healthcare profession: suppose you have a patient who would rather not undergo a minor operation and risk serious health consequences that could be easily avoided through this minor procedure. What is the right thing to do in this case? Is it best to simply passively accept the patient's wish—after all, consent, as we will see later on (chapter 6 of this book is indeed dedicated to consent within healthcare), is a fundamental requirement within healthcare? Or should one at least try to convince the patient by providing much more information and detail about the trivial nature of the procedure and the serious consequences of not intervening? Alternatively, should one put pressure on the patient or even try to coerce the patient into the procedure (say the patient is still very young or, on the other hand, senile)?

The point here goes beyond what is the best medical and ethical approach to this and countless other difficult cases that healthcare professionals face every day. Some of these cases may be easier to solve than others: in the one above, for example, it seems that providing more information would be the least that the doctor should do while coercion would appear to be going too far (except maybe for extreme circumstances that will have to do with the patient's state of mind). So this case is possibly not even that intractable—as opposed to, say, a case of breaking patient confidentiality in the hope of saving someone else's life.

Still, the point is not how easy or difficult these dilemmas are; the point is rather that the questions that need to be answered to decide what to do in such a case are not purely empirical questions: there are, it is obvious, medical considerations that are crucial to such a decision; but—and that is the main point here—answering all the relevant medical questions will still not tell you what to do in such a case; which is to say: purely medical questions, in the above case, do not exhaust all the relevant questions.[2]

And this is really, in a nutshell, my answer to our initial question: not all the questions and problems that healthcare professionals will have to address will be medical or, in broader terms, empirical ones; and that is why it is important—indeed, crucial—that healthcare professionals (and this also applies well beyond healthcare) engage with ethical and philosophical questions too. Basically, without those skills you will not be able to get the job done—it is as simple as that.

What other relevant questions are there, in such a case, beyond medical (and other empirical) questions? Here's one: when it comes to a patient's health, should we listen only to the doctor's expert opinion or also to the patient's wishes? This is not a medical question; neither is it another kind of empirical question, even though there is at least one sense in which answers to this question may be or become empirical: if they become the object of legislation.

If it is stipulated by law that the patient's wishes have to be taken into account, for example, then there would be an empirical answer to our question: namely, the law. Still, even in this particular—legal—sense of empirical questions and answers, the issue is unresolved: namely, what justifies a piece of legislation? What makes it a good law or one that it would be wrong to disobey?

Here, again, we may have to appeal to ethical considerations in order to justify legislation, which would again allow room for nonempirical questions (alternatively, one may just say that a law is just as long as it has been approved following appropriate procedures—say, voted in by a democratically elected parliament; but again it is easy to see here that some of these further issues are not easily resolved empirically, just think of the adjective 'appropriate' and the adverb 'democratically' above).

The basic point is, then, that there are questions that are not purely empirical and that are at the same time crucial to our decisions and to the problems that we face in real life: above we have identified at least two kinds of such questions, both of which are broadly philosophical. Some of these philosophical questions are purely theoretical; others are of a practical nature because they have more directly to do with deciding what to do.

Indeed, this will be a good way of thinking of philosophy and ethics—and philosophical and ethical questions—throughout: not as something distinct but rather in terms of ethical questions being one kind of philosophical question, the practical kind.

Here it is important not to mix up two different distinctions that we have made so far: on the one hand, we have started with a distinction between empirical and nonempirical (philosophical, if you like) questions; and now we have introduced the distinction between *practical* questions and *theoretical* questions. As it should be clear from our discussion so far, those are two different distinctions and, importantly, theoretical questions are not necessarily empirical and practical questions may also be empirical ones; indeed, here all combinations are possible.

There are theoretical questions of an empirical nature—a lot of questions within the basic natural sciences will belong to this group; and there are, as we have seen, theoretical questions that are not empirical, as the fundamental questions about existence or knowledge that we have discussed above. Similarly, there are practical questions that are not empirical, as the questions of ethics and moral philosophy.

There are also practical questions that are empirical though: suppose you are driving your friend home and you ask whether you should turn right or left at the next junction. That is a practical question: you want to know what to do there and then; but it is an empirical question too. Given what you are trying to achieve—driving your friend home—there will be better and worse answers to that question just as there will be shorter or longer routes (or more or less scenic routes, or ones with more or less traffic, or whatever).

We should keep these two distinctions separate then. Interestingly enough, medicine and healthcare transcend both of these two distinctions: the clinical nature of medical practice means that it is a practical as much as a theoretical discipline; and, as we have just seen, empirical questions and answers do not exhaust all the issues that are relevant in order to decide what to do as a doctor or other healthcare professional.

A side conceptual note before we move on: in thinking about the distinction between the theoretical and the practical, we should also say something about the concepts of medicine and healthcare, as our understanding and use of these concepts may very well depend on the practical-theoretical distinction. One could imagine, namely, the following two alternatives: on the one hand, medicine could be understood as one component of healthcare, which would then be the broader concept that also includes practices which are not necessarily medical ones: while probably nurses should count as being within medicine, it would not be implausible to think of care homes or also a lot of social work as, say, a nonmedical part of healthcare. But there is an alternative to this view of things: namely, that medicine is the theoretical head, if you like, and healthcare its practical arm. These distinctions may appear to be just another conceptual game but they could end up having significant implications to the way in which our health systems are organized.

Necessity and Objectivity

What does it mean that a question is or isn't empirical? It seems that we have been assuming a distinction, here, which could itself be taken to be controversial. In a basic and premature sense, we could say the following—and indeed something along these lines has been guiding us so far: empirical questions are those questions which science can at least hope to give an answer to.

This should not be taken to mean that these questions have already been answered by science nor that they have been answered correctly nor that they will ever be answered correctly by science; more modestly, it should for now be taken to mean that empirical questions are those that it is appropriate for science to try to answer—whether or not science will actually ever provide a satisfactory (true?) answer would then not be crucial to the empirical nature of the question.

If you are asking yourself how a question could ever be an empirical question if science will never manage to answer it (or answer it correctly), then it may be helpful to reflect upon the fact that science—as a human endeavour—is a limited enterprise in the basic sense that humans are cognitively limited in time, space, and capacities: that basically means that there may be questions which—in theory—are available for science to give an answer to but we will never get around to give or find the answer because of our limited cognitive capacities as humans.

Here again we should not confuse the attempt to make such a distinction between empirical and nonempirical questions and to ground it on what science can or cannot appropriately try to answer with the ability to neatly sort questions either under the 'empirical' heading or under the 'nonempirical' heading. This second task represents a further difficulty and there will be questions of which it will be hard to say where they belong and over which people will genuinely disagree.

CASE STUDY II: *The Existence of God*

Think of the following question: does god exist? Remember, the point here is not to answer the question but merely to establish whether this question is an empirical one. This last point is important because we could imagine quite a few possibilities:

A) god exists and the question of its existence is an empirical question;
B) god exists and the question of its existence is not an empirical question;
C) god does not exist and the question of its existence is an empirical question;
D) god does not exist and the question of its existence is not an empirical question.

There are probably more alternatives than the four above (agnosticism, for example—or the meaninglessness of the question) but I will stick to the ones above for now.

It is probably fair to say that most if not all monotheistic religions hold (B) rather than (A) and take it to be very important—indeed, all-important—that (B) rather than (A) is the case. Here we can't go into any theological detail but the basic point is that the existence of god is supposed to be necessary rather than contingent, so the standard religious claim will not be merely that: god exists; it will rather be the stronger claim that: god necessarily exists.

It is consistent with the former claim but not with the latter claim that god may have not existed—that's the crucial difference and that's the reason why most if not all religions go for the latter rather than the former; and indeed god would provide even less explanation than it may do now within religious worldviews if its existence were a mere fact of empirical contingence; god could not, for example—to go back to a question we have already mentioned—even begin to answer the question of why being rather than nothing if its very existence was contingent.

The philosophical debate over the existence of god recognizes this and provides *a priori* arguments and counterarguments for or against the existence of god: just to mention two famous ones, the *ontological argument* tries to show that god must, by definition, exist; while the *argument from evil* tries to show that god cannot exist for the simple reason that its existence would imply a contradiction between its benevolent, all-powerful and omniscient nature on the one hand and the existence of evil on the other hand.[3]

Both those arguments, despite aiming at opposing conclusions, share the fact of not being contingent ones, as the ontological argument aims to show not just that god exists but that god *necessarily* exists and the argument from evil aims to show not just that god does not exist but that god *cannot* exist—namely that its nonexistence is again a necessity.[4]

Even within a naturalistic worldview, the difference between (C) and (D) is possibly as important as the difference between (A) and (B) will be within a religious worldview. This is because only (C) allows for scientific evidence or scientific method more in general to have anything to say about the existence or, rather, nonexistence of god. Option (D), on the other hand, puts the nonexistence of god beyond science; (D) may, in this sense, seem the strongest option but it is—symmetrically with (B)—one that makes science powerless as to the question of god—the very approach that most religions favour. The argument from evil that we have just encountered would then be an argument in support of (D) rather than (C), for example; just as the ontological argument would be an argument in support of (B) rather than (A).

This is not the place to entertain the question of god in any further detail: it has rather been a vehicle to better understand talk of empirical and nonempirical questions. At the same time, though, we now have at least three further distinctions that must be added to the two we have already identified:

I. empirical and nonempirical
II. theoretical and practical
III. necessary and contingent
IV. objective and subjective
V. *a priori* and *a posteriori*[5]

We have already shown the difference between (I) and (II); but what about those new ones, especially as with the question of the existence of god we seem to have used interchangeably (I) and (III). Each of these five distinctions has, alone, been the subject of countless books over, at least, the last three millennia. So it is not really my place, here, to hope to give any satisfactory—let alone complete—account of them.

What I will try to do, much more minimally, is to point out some important differences between these distinctions, just in the spirit in which we have already explained how not to confuse (I) with (II) since, in that particular case, all four combinations are possible.

Very broadly speaking—which really means cutting some corners—we may be allowed to, for now, throw together (I), (III), and (V) while pointing out the similarities and overlaps between empirical, contingent, and *a posteriori* on the one side and necessary, *a priori* and nonempirical on the other side. This will do for now while we rather concentrate on distinguishing those from the distinction between objective and subjective, which cuts across and therefore should be kept separate.

It would be admittedly tempting to simply take empirical questions and answers (more generally we should really talk about statements and propositions) to be objective ones and the remaining nonempirical statements to be subjective statements. Preferences provide us with a good example here: whether a tiger is quicker than a lion is an empirical question and, accordingly, there will be an objective answer to this question; whether tigers are more beautiful animals than lions seems to be, on the other hand, a question that cannot be settled empirically and that will not have an objective answer.

There may be room for meaningful and maybe even interesting debate about whether, aesthetically, lions or tigers are preferable—but it is difficult to imagine an objective answer to this question (even though, having said that, we should not rule it out altogether: there may be a canon against which such debate is conducted and there may be an objective answer as to whether, given that aesthetic canon, a tiger is to be preferable to a lion).

The fact that empirical questions and objective answers can be linked as above does not mean, though, that we are looking at one and the same distinction when we take (I) and (IV). That is because there is at least logical room for objective truths that are not empirical truths. Here is an example: mathematical truths are objective truths but they are not empirical truths in any standard sense; it is both objectively and necessarily true that two plus three equals five but this truth does not depend on any facts—natural or empirical facts—about our world.[6]

We have seen this point earlier as we discussed the idea of necessary versus contingent facts, such as the existence of god. If two plus three equals five is a necessary truth, then it is not a contingent truth, differently from the contingent truth that there are more than seven fruits on my table as I write this. There could have been fewer than seven fruits on my table this morning—it would have just taken for the world to have been very slightly different, as in a world where I would have eaten more fruit yesterday or a world where I would have bought less fruit or something along these lines.

We cannot say the same about mathematical truths, and that is why they are not contingent. But—and that's the interesting bit here—while the number of fruits on my table this morning and two plus three equals five differ in terms of contingency, they share objectivity. It is an objective fact that there are more than seven fruits on my table this morning just as it is an objective fact that two plus three equals five.

These objective facts must, in turn, be distinguished from subjective facts. Here there is a further complication: we may speak of subjective facts to talk about facts regarding our mental life, for example—or indeed our preferences. I may desire to run faster than a tiger or I may like lions better than I like tigers or I may believe that tigers are quicker than lions; those are subjective facts in the sense that they are facts about me that have no further claim than expressing something about my preferences, desires, or beliefs.

CASE STUDY III: *Lions vs. Tigers*

Still, while my belief that tigers are quicker than lions should not be confused with the fact of the matter as to whether members of the one species tend to be quicker than members of the other species (a quick Internet search, by the way, does appear to confirm that tigers tend to have a significant advantage over lions with regard to both agility and physical strength), both are objective in the sense that, if I believe that tigers are quicker than lions, then it is an objective fact that I have a belief with that content; similarly, if it is scientifically proven that tigers are faster, stronger (or whatever) than lions, then it is an objective fact that this is so.

Those objective facts have different contents obviously, because one is about me while the other is about tigers and lions, but that does not make the facts about my beliefs any less objective; even though they will clearly have a much narrower scope as they will say nothing about what others think nor about whether my belief is actually true.

Subjectivity

Where does this leave subjectivity? There are at least two further senses of 'subjective' that we should identify apart from the already discussed sense of subjective as in *the subject's*, as for my belief that tigers are faster than lions as opposed to the matter of fact on the issue.

CASE STUDY IV: *Stracciatella Ice Cream*

Some content may be thought to be intrinsically subjective, as with ice cream preferences. Take, on the one hand, my preference for stracciatella over, say, strawberry and on the other hand my belief that tigers are faster than lions. While in the latter case there is a fact of the matter as to whether tigers are indeed faster than lions, and therefore there is a fact of the matter as to the truth or falsity of my belief—even though that fact is clearly independent of my beliefs on the matter—in the former case there does not seem to be any equivalent fact of the matter as to the relative or absolute merits of stracciatella and strawberry. So the taste of stracciatella is not like the speed of lions: it cannot, if you like, be measured.[7]

This means that the subjectivity of my taste for stracciatella goes beyond the fact that it is *my* taste, as with *my* belief that tigers are faster than lions. And still even here we ought to recognize that the fact that I prefer stracciatella to strawberry is an objective fact about my preferences the same way in which the fact that I believe that tigers are faster than lions is an objective fact about my beliefs.

The other sense of subjective is more difficult to pin down: it has to do with the mind and its peculiar perspective. The mental, after all, is unique in both being *in* the world and being *about* the world—indeed, in having a perspective in the first place. A lot has been written about the 'aboutness' of the mental and so-called mental content but here I just want to emphasize this further possible sense of subjective and subjectivity, namely the intrinsically irreducible character of the mind's perspective on the world.

Identifying—even in concrete terms—the content of a perception, belief, or desire is, after all, possible: it may be about tigers just as much as it may be about stracciatella. And those things are real. But—to quote Thomas Nagel—what is it like to love a tiger? What is it like to prefer a tiger to a lion or stracciatella to strawberry? Specifically, what is it like for me (or for you) to have such a preference? And so on.

This perspective—often also referred to as phenomenal character—of experience (whether human or maybe also animal or even alien) is not as concrete as tigers or stracciatella; and if it is in any meaningful sense subjective, it is subjective in a different way from the other senses of subjectivity that we have identified above.

The supposed subjectivity of the mental is not something that you should take as a given: indeed, whether some form of naturalism or materialism is true of the mental is a crucial unresolved question in contemporary philosophy of mind, so I don't want to give the impression that this—or indeed much of anything else—is settled. If you are starting to wonder why all this talk of the mind is at all relevant to healthcare, just think of the complicated issue of the role and status of mental health within healthcare; acknowledging the importance of mental health and its parity with other health conditions may at least in part depend on a good understanding of the mind and its relationship with brain, body and environment.

The mind is important also because it raises one more of the great questions of humanity: the problem of liberty and causation. In a nutshell: how can there be any freedom—of will and of action—if everything that we think and do is causally determined? And if it isn't—namely if the universe is not in itself causally closed, say because the mind does not follow the rules of causation—aren't we violating one of the fundamental principles upon which our scientific method is based?

This is the view that is often referred to as *determinism* or causal determinism, that has historically been taken to make a difference to the question of whether we have free will and the question of whether we can ever be morally responsible for what we do (more on responsibility in chapter 8).

The question is closely related to the previous one about the nature of the mind: on the one hand, we would like to say that the mind, being part of everything else (the universe, if you like), follows the laws that govern everything else, namely the laws of nature. If the causal closure of the universe is one of these laws and if the mind is part of it, then the mind would also be subject to the laws of causation, which imply that any state of the universe is completely causally determined by a previous state of the universe.

This appears to have implications for free will and free action, at least intuitively—because it would mean that our desires, beliefs, intentions and emotions—just to cite a few states of the mind—are themselves subject to this causal determination. Take the following example: as I checked the weather report this morning, I decided that it was dry enough—no rain was forecast—to go running, so I formed the intention to go running; acting on that intention, I later went for a run.

The causal closure of the universe means that all the elements in that decision-making process were causally determined by a previous state of the universe. That means that the way in which the universe was on, say, the third of September 1958 determined the way the universe was at any future moment in time, including the moment in which I checked the weather report, the moment in which I decided to go running, and the moment in which I went for a run.

There has always been a very lively debate about these issues, but the above means, at least at first glance, that when I decided to go for a run I could not have not decided to go for a run—that is just what it means for my decision to have been causally determined by previous states of the universe going back before I or my ancestors were born. Additionally, these issues have been historically taken to have consequences for the idea of moral responsibility: if when I decided to go for a run I could not have not decided to go for a run, am I responsible for having gone for a run (especially given that both my intention and my action are supposed to be causally determined)?

Here again we don't have the time to go into more details (again see chapter 8 for an in-depth discussion of responsibility), but it will suffice to notice that we are once more faced with questions that rather than being scientific questions, they are questions *about* science in the first place—and this alone should be enough to make us suspect that we need something more; possibly, indeed, philosophy.

We can now see that another obvious candidate for a nonempirical question has been lurking in the background all this time: namely, the basic issue of whether a question can be settled empirically or not. 'Are we inevitably all going to die?' is a question that we should really regard as empirical but over which some people may disagree on either religious grounds or—misguided—futuristic ambitions of life extension. And indeed—depending on the definition of death—at least those religiously motivated doubts may even be coherent if, say, one postulates an afterlife. As we have seen, the question over the existence of god is one where actually a lot of the debate does not turn over whether a positive or negative answer is defensible, but rather on the nature of the question and whether empirical evidence has any role to play in answering it.

Here there is one possible confusion that should be avoided: conceptual matters of definition and meaning will be relevant to all questions, whether they are empirical or not—see the above points about the definition of something as concrete as 'death' or as abstract as 'god': how these concepts work and what their properties are is clearly crucial but it should not be taken to mean that no question can be settled empirically. It is rather that some issues are just a matter of definition, such as two plus three equals five, while other issues are not just a matter of definition.

Why is any of this worth your time anyway, you may ask? A first answer to this question is what we have been delivering so far: namely, some questions cannot be resolved purely empirically but that does not mean that they are not important, both theoretically and practically, as we have seen. Here we have tried to make a start in showing what these questions may be and what it means that they cannot be answered empirically. In the next chapter, our focus will be on a particular kind of nonempirical questions, namely ethical and moral ones.

Summary

In this chapter, we have discussed the role of philosophical questions within healthcare: we have argued that not all interesting questions are empirical questions and that, even within healthcare, not all medical questions are empirical questions—so philosophy's basic contribution is to address the other important questions which cannot be settled empirically. We have briefly discussed the example of the question of the existence of god to show that not all important questions are necessarily empirical questions. On top of the distinction between empirical questions and questions that cannot be settled empirically, we have also distinguished between theoretical questions and practical questions and between objective and subjective answers. In the next chapter, we will use these distinctions in order to introduce a particular set of questions which are practical but not, on the face of it, empirical: moral or ethical questions.

Notes

1. Here it may be worth noting that one of the most popular views in the philosophy of mind today, often referred to as the *extended mind* hypothesis (going back to Andy Clark and David Chalmers) would plausibly speak against pointing your index finger towards your head as the mind, according to this view, is supposed to be extended even beyond our body to tools and the environment around us.

2. Note that here we may not even be able to say that those questions are not 'medical' questions; it is not implausible to define medical questions as questions whose answers are important for doctors to do their job well; under such definitions, a lot of medical questions will not be empirical ones and a lot of the moral issues that healthcare professionals have to deal with will qualify as 'medical' questions. But not much turns on the definition of 'medical' once we have accepted the broader point about there being non-empirical questions worth asking and answering.

3. If you are interested in finding out more about these issues, a great place to start is the SEP article on *Ontological Arguments*, freely available online here: https://plato.stanford.edu/entries/ontological-arguments/.

4. Admittedly, the argument from evil has at least one empirical premise, namely the premise that: there is evil in this world.

5. To avoid further complication, here I am disregarding a further distinction which would otherwise be both important and relevant, namely the distinction analytic/synthetic. The standard case of an analytic sentence would be 'all bachelors are unmarried', true by definition, so to speak.

6. For a classic discussion of this, see Willard Van Orman Quine's 'Two Dogmas of Empiricism', *The Philosophical Review* 60, no. 1 (1951): 20–43.

7. This is not to be confused with my belief about my preferences: I may have a belief that I prefer stracciatella over strawberry, and that belief my function just like my belief that tigers are faster than lions; namely, if tigers are indeed faster than lions, then my belief of that content is true; and if I indeed prefer stracciatella over strawberry, then my

belief of that content is also true. This question is, though, a separate one from the question of whether there is a fact of the matter about the relative culinary merits of stracciatella over strawberry—there very likely is not; which is what distinguishes the relative culinary merits of stracciatella over strawberry from the relative merits of tigers over lions in terms of speed—where there is indeed a fact of the matter.

CHAPTER TWO

Right and Wrong

From Moral Objectivity to Relativism

Moral and ethical questions are one crucial example of questions that cannot be settled empirically. At the same time, ethical and moral questions are—as we have seen—practical questions in the sense that they are about what one should do. They are, in this sense, urgent. And their practical nature makes them particularly important not especially for philosophers, actually, but exactly for those that can make a difference (and *have* to make a difference) in the real world, like for example doctors, other healthcare professionals, and those in other strategic professions.

Now we have the instruments to say a bit more about the nature of ethical and moral questions, starting from what we have achieved so far: namely that such questions are practical but not empirical but that this does not mean that the relevant answers cannot be thought to be, possibly, objective.

CASE STUDY I: Mary's Secret

Take the following moral judgment: 'Lisa should not have told Mary's secret to Kate even though it greatly helped Rosa'. Or take the following general moral principle: 'killing children can never be justified'.[1] About these two statements we can ask the following question: do you agree with the statements? We can also ask a different question: are the statements true? Those two questions are obviously different but both are plausible questions to ask about the moral statements above.

This may seem like we have just stated the obvious but we can see that there is something to learn from it actually: compare the above statements with statements such as, for example, 'stracciatella tastes better than strawberry'. Now we can see that, of this latter statement, it makes sense only to ask the question about whether we agree with it but we cannot really meaningfully ask the question of whether the statement is true (as we have seen previously, a different story in this context would be the statement 'stracciatella tastes to Ezio better than strawberry').

So we have identified an important difference between, on the one hand, moral statements—whether particular ones like the example of Marie and Rose or general ones like the killing children example—and, on the other hand, preferences such as culinary ones (broader aesthetic preferences such as artistic ones may be somewhere in between but we can't go into that now). This difference is important because it prevents us from straightforwardly categorizing moral statements as subjective ones like simple culinary preferences.

Both moral judgements and culinary preferences, though, must be distinguished from basic descriptive statements such as, to take something we have already used, the proposition 'there are more than seven fruits on my table'. What is the difference? After all, of this latter statement we can also ask whether people agree with it and we can certainly ask whether it is true or false. In this respect, then, this latter statement should belong together with moral judgments and it would have to be distinguished from culinary preferences.

At the same time, though, there seems to be an obvious difference between our moral judgments and a statement of fact such as 'there are more than seven fruits on my table'. What is this supposedly obvious difference? We have already ruled out taking the shortcut of just saying that the latter is objective while the former is purely subjective; even if it were, it would seem to be subjective in an importantly different way from how culinary preferences are thought to be subjective, as we have just shown.

Here we may go back to the talk of empirical verifiability that we used at the start: we can find out whether or not there are more than seven fruits of my table. But can we find out whether or not Lisa should have told Marie's secret? What would it even mean to find out whether killing children cannot be justified? So now we see, at least superficially, an obvious difference again between moral judgements and statements of facts like the number of fruits on my table.

We have identified, then, at least three kinds of judgments:

1) judgments of taste like culinary ones;
2) moral judgments;
3) judgments of fact.

Things could be made even more complicated by adding the already referred to examples from mathematics, which may deserve a further category, as we have seen. But I think the above three will be enough for now.

What (1) and (2) have in common is that they are not empirically verifiable while what (2) and (3) have in common is that we can meaningfully ask whether those judgments are true, even though what makes them true or false may be significantly different in each case.

If (2) and (3) have in common that we can genuinely ask the question of whether one agrees with the statements and also have in common that we can genuinely ask the question of whether the statements are true, what difference is there at all between the two?

The Ontological and the Epistemological

Here we can certainly go back to the talk of empirical verifiability, but in that respect the time has come to introduce a further distinction, between

A) ontological questions; and
B) epistemological questions.

We need this distinction because saying that (2) and (3) are different in terms of the way in which they can be verified says something about their epistemological status but not about their ontological status. Put in another way, the question of verifiability has to do with how we can *know* that a statement is true or false; it is not about *whether* the statement is true or false.

More generally, ontological questions are questions about what there is while epistemological questions are questions about what we can know; the point of making the distinction in the first place is that the fact that we do not or cannot know something does not itself imply that the thing does not exist—again, that does not follow exactly because of the unwarranted move between the two levels, from an epistemological premise to an ontological conclusion.

The distinction between epistemological questions and ontological questions also allows us to see an underestimated difference which is already within (2) alone; moral judgments can be very different from each other. Take the example of Mary's secret and compare it with the example of the principle against killing children: their ontological status appears to be similar; neither of them is empirical and both of them have at least the ambition of objectivity—whether that can be fulfilled or not is a different matter.

When we look at the two moral judgments from an epistemological point of view, though, we see that—in terms of knowing the truth of these judgments—the difference may be significant; and that's because the former moral judgment (the one about Mary's secret) is *particular* while the other one is *general* (not to be confused with *universal*, more on this later).

This is a simple point: the particular moral judgment is about a specific historical or fictional action or event and it judges that particular action or event; what it says may have the scope to be applicable to relevantly similar actions or events but it is about that particular one. While the general principle against killing children does not refer to any specific historical or fictional case but to a category of cases; indeed, to any case which has the property of 'killing children'.[2]

The difference between particular and general moral judgments is of some consequence, as it may affect the truth of those judgments and also our knowledge of them, especially in terms of warrant/justification. The first difference is just that even if moral judgments may be true, it will be easier for particular moral judgments to be true than for general moral judgments. Indeed, it is at least possible to imagine a moral system in which some particular judgments are true but no general judgments are true (philosophers often refer to Jonathan Dancy's *particularism* in this context[3]).

The second difference is a question of justification, and it is related to the first: it may be easier to justify a particular moral judgment than to justify a general one, as it will be always possible to come up with objections and counterexamples against something with that level of generality and that is not necessarily the case with particular moral judgments. Having looked at these possible differences within (2), let us now return to the question of the difference between (2) and (3), which is, I dare say, more important to our purposes.

Having distinguished between the ontological level and the epistemological level, we can see that (2) and (3) may be different from an epistemological point of view but that does not mean or imply any difference at the ontological level—which is, if you like, the same reason why we said that we could not assume that nonempirical questions could not have objective answers.

Still we are left with the old question: what is the difference between moral judgments and judgments of fact? One traditional way of distinguishing between these two is by saying that the latter are *descriptive* statements while the former are *normative* statements. Let me now explain this further distinction (just the sheer number of distinctions that I have introduced so far should tell you something about the nature of philosophy, by the way).

The idea is that descriptive statements fulfil a different task than the one that normative statements are supposed to fulfil: the former tell us how the world *is* while the latter tell us how the world *should* be. Think again about our examples: to say that there are more than seven fruits on my table is one of countless ways in which we describe the way in which the world actually is. It could have easily been different but, as it turns out, it is such that there are more than seven fruits on the table.

This alone does not say anything at all about the speaker's preferences towards this state of affairs: whether the speaker would have preferred fewer fruits on the table, say. Nor does the statement say anything about the value of this state of affairs beyond the speaker's preferences. The statement is, if you like, neutral—exactly in virtue of the fact that it is merely descriptive.

Now this cannot be said of normative statements: when we say that Lisa should not have told Marie's secret to Kate, we do implicitly say something about how the world is—namely that Lisa did tell Marie's secret to Kate—but crucially we also add some value—in this case negative value—to this statement. So the statement is not neutral; and this is because the statement does not simply describe the way in which the world happens to be but it actually also expresses a preference as to the way the world *should* have actually been: the action in question should not have been performed.

This is, then, the normative character of moral judgments: they appeal to a norm to express a value preference about the way things should have been. Here the implicit norm—we may suppose—has something to do with keeping secrets and promises more in general. And the idea is that the norm—and its application to this concrete example—makes what Lisa did wrong or anyway morally problematic—where 'wrong' here (and throughout if not explicitly specified) means 'morally wrong'.

Show Me the Mo . . . rals

This may sound all too technical, at least as long as it does not answer the following simple question: if someone does not agree (indeed, does not *see*) that there are more than seven fruits on the table, I can simply *show* them that there are more than seven fruits on the table—sure, the ability to count complicates this, but one could just as easily take an example with just one single fruit. But imagine someone who does not agree that Lisa should not have told Marie's secret to Kate. How do I show them that my moral judgment is true? How do I show them that I am right?

This is, after all, important—we have already agreed that moral judgments, whatever they are, function differently, at least in our language if not beyond it, from simple matters of culinary taste. When it comes to ethics, then, the truth of moral judgements is important while, at the same time, we cannot just show it by reference to the real world, it seems. This is, again, for the simple reason that normative statements have this added value which makes them difficult to reduce to descriptive statements, the truth or falsity of which we can, at least in principle, show or demonstrate.

The question could be thought to be the relatively-speaking more minor one of how to deal with and solve moral disagreement; this is indeed an important question in its own right but much more is at stake here. What is at stake is, first, whether moral judgments can even be true or false; yes, we may speak as if they were in some sense true or false—as opposed to culinary preferences—but is it really so?

Secondly, even if we can show that they are true or false in some significant sense, there is the further question of how to show or demonstrate their truth or falsity, since it is unlikely that—if moral judgments are indeed true or false—they will be self-evidently so. After all, disagreement on matters of value is a fact of our world. It is one that—importantly—does not imply that there is no underlying truth to any of this; but still, the mere fact that there is disagreement makes the epistemological question just as pressing as the ontological one.

CASE STUDY II: *Torture Works (sic.)*

So we are left with the big question—and it is a pressing one not just theoretically but also practically, given widespread moral disagreement not just about details but about some fundamental human questions; just think of Donald Trump's first interview as president of the United States, when he went on record saying that 'torture works'.

The first thing we should look at, in tackling this big question of moral objectivity, is what kind of objectivity we are even looking for—as we will see in a moment, this is no trivial matter. On the face of it, we may think that the best objectivity one could ask for—when it comes to ethics and moral questions—is the objectivity of nature and science. If we could just *prove* our moral judgments and values! This wish is understandable but, I will argue, misguided.

Actually, the argument is a version of one that we have already encountered. Remember what we said about religions: they are mostly not interested in proving, empirically, the existence of god—think of the concept of faith, for example; and the reason for that is, as we said, that they don't just want god to exist, they want god to exist noncontingently, independently of the contingent facts of the natural world. This is an important distinction also when it comes to moral objectivity.

Let us take the example of torture. When we say that torture is wrong and we mean for that moral judgement about torture to have an objective scope which goes beyond mere expression of our attitude towards torture, we are saying something more than just describing widespread attitudes towards torture; indeed, we are saying that torture is wrong independently of how people actually judge torture to be—that is the all point of the judgement being objective, that its truth or falsity is independent of people's beliefs, similarly to the way in which the judgment that our planet is not flat is true independently of people's beliefs about the flatness of our planet and indeed has always been true even at times when nobody believed that our planet was not flat.

So far the similarity with facts from the empirical sciences—again, there is similarity in virtue of both empirical and moral judgments having objective *scope* (here the best word is really the German *anspruch*; so think of 'scope' in terms of 'claim', 'aspiration'). But there is obviously a difference: we want to say, of the roundish form of our earth, that it could have also been flat: it is just a contingent empirical fact that it happens to not be flat, there is no necessity there.

The same does not apply to moral judgment: so we don't want to say of torture that it is wrong but that it could have also been right or justified. If torture is wrong, it is necessarily so. A helpful way of formulating this is in conceptual terms: torture would not be torture if it were not wrong, that is what we are saying when we say that it is wrong. But we have to be careful with this conceptual talk, because of many practices it is not clear that wrongness necessarily belongs to them even if we do judge them wrong.

This talk of noncontingent objectivity, by the way, should not be understood in terms of making moral judgement wholly independent of the reality on the ground, so to speak. That people suffer tremendous physical and psychological pain when they are tortured is obviously one of the reasons why torture is wrong. On the other hand, we also need to be careful with equating the wrongness of torture with such 'measurables' like pain for the simple reason that it would beg the question of the wrongness of pain.

You may be asking yourself the following question now: if moral judgement is supposed to be both objectively true and nonempirically so, where are truth and objectivity coming from, if they are not coming from us—the people—and nor are they coming from the natural world? Now that we have distinguished between ontology and epistemology, we can see that that is just another version—the ontological version if you like—of our original hard question of how we prove that a moral judgement is true or false and demonstrate it to those that disagree. So, where do moral truths come from if they are to be noncontingent?

CASE STUDY III: *God, Again . . .*

One obvious candidate is god. God, if it existed, would have exactly the noncontingent qualities needed for moral judgment. Before briefly presenting a classic argument—from Plato—against the idea of deriving morality from god, I want to point out a preliminary difficulty with this approach. The truth of moral judgment has practical implications just in virtue of the practical nature of moral judgment. If the idea of appealing to god is an epistemological idea of providing justification for moral judgement, then the fact that, as most religions maintain, the existence of god is a matter of faith rather than belief, is not a very promising starting point for morality. Moral judgement may not be supposed to be contingent, but that ought not to mean that moral arguments should just be a matter of faith—not in principle anyway.

So faith is a problem, particularly when it comes to the justification of moral judgment. Still, why not appeal to god's authority when it comes to the origins of moral truths? This option is often referred to as *divine command theory* for, well, obvious reasons. And there is a classic argument against it in Plato's *Euthyphro* (that's one of Plato's dialogues, taking its name from Socrates' sparring partner); the argument itself is normally referred to accordingly as the *Euthyphro Dilemma* and it originates in the following question that Socrates poses to Euthyphro: 'Consider the following point: is the holy approved by the gods because it's holy, or is it holy because it's approved?' (10a).[4]

Here divine command theorists are presented with two options: either they can reply that—reformulating in terms that we have been using—god approves of some action because it is right or they can reply that some action is right because god approves of it. Both options are problematic—that's why it's a dilemma. The first option—god approves of an action because it is morally right—flies in the face of the whole project under examination here of grounding morality with god because it makes morality independent of god to say that god approves of an action because it is, independently of god itself that is, right. This would also have further problems in terms of god omnipotence as it suggests that god is not the ultimate tribunal—but this last point is not crucial for our purposes.

The main problem with this first option is simply that if the point of the divine command theory is to appeal to god's authority, then it is contradictory to say that god approves of something because it is right independently of its approval. This leaves us with the other option, according to which an action is right because god approves of it—namely, god makes that action right by approving of it. This is more in line with the project of the divine command theory but it has other problems: mostly, that morality would become arbitrary and contingent to god's approval. Only what is approved by god is right and, supposedly, what is disapproved by god is wrong.

But what if god approved wrong things and disapproved right things? And indeed religious texts are full of nasty people and actions that god apparently approves of or at least does not condemn—reflecting the historical nature of these supposedly holy texts, obviously. Here we should note that the mere fact that religious texts are full of unethical people and actions is no argument against the second option according to which something is right because god approves of it, for the simple reason that religious texts may themselves be wrong about god's intentions and beliefs—remember here again the distinction between epistemology and ontology, in this case between what god intends and our knowledge of god's intentions.

The example of religious texts then is rather an illustration of the problem rather than itself a problem: the problem is that according to the second option morality would in the end be arbitrary and contingent, albeit contingent upon a being which is itself meant to be infallible. So one classic reply to arguments against the second option is to say that god could not approve wrong actions—exactly because of its infallibility. But it is difficult to say how this reply makes any progress on the original dilemma, as the definition of 'wrong action' is exactly what we were looking for in the first place.[5]

So god's out—at least as a source of morality, and that's without having had to appeal to classic arguments against its benevolence (or existence) like the argument from evil that we have encountered in chapter 1. We are, in a certain way, back where we started: on the one hand, we want to say that torture is morally wrong and that this is objectively so, independently of what Trump and his supporters may say or believe; on the other hand, given that the judgement that 'torture is wrong' is a normative one, its truth cannot depend simply on matters of fact, not in any empirical sense of fact anyway.

I can imagine here the reader becoming impatient in at least two different respects: on the one hand, some readers may point out that we should just start enunciating the many good arguments for the claim that torture is indeed wrong. At the other end of the spectrum, someone could say that I have been disregarding, so far, an obvious alternative, namely that moral judgements such as 'torture is wrong' are simply not to be spoken of in terms of objective truth because that's just not the way morality works.

Meta-ethics

Those two points are actually related in the following way: both can be taken to be reminders of the need to introduce one more distinction—and I am afraid I am far from being in a position to promise that this is going to be the last one:

- meta-ethics
- normative ethics

There are different kinds of questions that one may ask about a statement such as 'torture is wrong'—and that, just to be clear, also applies to a particular statement involving torture, so that the point I am about to make does not hinge on the particular–general distinction that we have discussed:

1) it is possible to inquire about the *meaning* of the statement 'torture is wrong';

2) it is also possible to inquire *whether* the statement 'torture is wrong' is true (or false);
3) and it is possible to inquire *why* the statement 'torture is wrong' is true (or false).

It has become commonplace in philosophy to distinguish between what are now two distinct disciplines: *meta-ethics* deals with questions such as (1) while *normative ethics* deals with questions such as (3)—more about (2) in a moment. Within the former, we find theories about the meaning (and nature, if you like) of ethical statements or judgements; in the latter we find normative theories that tell us which actions are right and wrong and why they are right or wrong.

This distinction allows you to see that up until now we have hardly taken up any normative ethics and we have pretty much asked only meta-ethical questions about the meaning and nature of moral judgement. As those issues are independent of each other to a great extent, we will keep this structure and deal with normative ethical questions from the next chapter—the rest of this chapter will conclude our discussion of what we now know is called meta-ethics.

That is why we will not engage with normative arguments about why torture is wrong or whether torture 'works' (whatever that's supposed to mean, Mr. President) and other similar debates: we first need to understand the meaning of the statement 'torture is wrong'. As promised, though, a note on (2), the question of truth. Whether moral judgment in general can ever be true is a meta-ethical question; while whether a specific moral judgement like 'torture is wrong' is indeed true or false is a normative question and the answer will depend on which normative theory one endorses.

Speaking of truth is therefore not very helpful in making the distinction between meta-ethics and normative ethics; it is easier to think in terms of meta-ethics as the discipline that looks at the question of the meaning of moral judgment and of normative ethics as the discipline that looks at the question of the justification of moral judgement(s).

Of the two earlier complaints we now see that the one about the many good arguments for the wrongness of torture is premature: that is an issue in normative ethics that does not belong here. The other complaint, though, was spot on: moral objectivity is an open question in meta-ethics and we cannot simply assume it, as we will see below.

Let us start from the basic question of what it means to say that 'torture is wrong'. So-called noncognitivists would say that a moral judgement such as 'torture is wrong' should be understood as equivalent to 'I am against torture'; as we have already discussed in comparing moral judgement to aesthetic or culinary judgement, this difference is important and not merely technical.

The scope of what you are saying if you are only saying (indeed, if what you can say only ever is) that you are against torture is much more limited than what the grammatical structure of a statement like 'torture is wrong' would at first glance suggest—namely that I am not just expressing my view on torture but that I am saying something about torture which is applicable beyond my own perspective.

There is a simple way of understanding the difference between 'I am against torture' and 'torture is wrong': compare these two statements with Trump's 'torture works' (which, we may assume, is his way of saying that torture is not wrong). The statement 'torture is not wrong' is not compatible with the statement 'torture is wrong' but it is compatible with the statement 'S is against torture' as only the former statement—'torture is wrong'—contradicts 'torture is not wrong'.

Imagine two people having the following—very sterile, I will admit—dialogue:

O: 'Torture is unethical'.
T: 'You are wrong: torture is not unethical'.
O: 'No, you are wrong: torture is unethical'.

Now translate this dialogue in noncognitivist terms and you obtain:

O: 'I am against torture'.
T: 'You are wrong: I am not against torture'.
O: 'No, you are wrong: I am against torture'.

You can easily see that, banal as it is, the first version of the dialogue makes sense: those two people are talking to each other. They are disagreeing, but they are communicating and doing so successfully. The latter dialogue is, on the other hand, a mess, as T takes herself to be contradicting O with her reply while her reply is obviously not contradicting O, rather it is stating something which is different but compatible with what O is saying: namely that T, differently from O, is not against torture. And then O goes on to make exactly the same mistake as T. This little artificial dialogue was just a quick way to show the consequences of these differences in meaning.

The disagreement between cognitivists and noncognitivists is, then, first of all, a disagreement about how we speak about morality: not, clearly, about the words we use—as that would be an empirical disagreement—but rather about the meaning of those words. The implication is that, according to noncognitivists, we cannot even express moral objectivity, not beyond the narrow objectivity of it being the case that someone holds a certain moral preference.

It is now easy to see that this has consequences for the very possibility of moral judgment being true or false. When we think of the truth of a judgement like 'torture is wrong' or of the falsity of Trump's claim that 'torture works', we normally do not think that the only sense in which such statement may even be true is that it is true that the speaker of 'torture is wrong' disapproves of torture or that it is true that Trump approves of torture. Indeed, Trump uttering 'torture works' does at least conventionally imply that Trump approves of torture; but, again, we would normally understand Trump to be saying more than just something about his attitude or desire—we would normally take him to express a belief about the value of torture.

Similarly, the speaker of 'torture is wrong' will, with that utterance, indeed conventionally imply that she disapproves of torture but if we say that the speaker has spoken the truth we would normally not be meaning that she has been truthful about her disapproval but that her statement about torture is true in a more substantial or robust sense.

Let me say one more thing about noncognitivism and the truth of moral judgements. What are the truth conditions of a statement such as 'torture is wrong'? Cognitivists will insist that these truth conditions have something to do with the nature of torture, of which the property wrongness is being predicated. This is supposed to work—at least in theory—just in the same way as the statement 'the car is red' works; the statement is true if and only if the car is indeed red; otherwise it is false. In the same way, 'torture is wrong' is true, according to cognitivists, if and only if torture is indeed wrong.

The truth conditions of the statement 'torture is wrong' will be very different for noncognitivists though, because they will not have anything to do with torture but rather will depend on whether the speaker approves or disapproves of torture, so that according to a noncognitivist the statement is true if and only if the speaker disapproves of torture. Visualizing this will make the difference obvious:

COGNITIVIST: ‘torture is wrong’ is true if and only if *torture is indeed wrong*;

NONCOGNITIVIST: ‘torture is wrong’ is true if and only if *the speaker disapproves of torture*.

Summing up, it looks as though we normally speak as if moral judgement was meant to have some objectivity and truth; on the other hand, though, since moral judgements are not merely descriptive, establishing their truth is challenging, as we have now seen from many perspectives. I would now like to conclude this chapter by discussing what could be considered to be a compromise position between these two difficulties: *relativism*.

Moral Relativism

If a man rapes a woman in, say, Denmark (and if he is caught, which does not happen often enough), the man is punished. If a man rapes a woman in Saudi Arabia, it is the woman who is punished.[6]

CASE STUDY IV: *Rape Culture*

Diversity is not always a good thing. Sometimes, like with the case above, it is very clear that one of the practices is unacceptable. But things are not always that simple. Think of the following two alternative cases:

- let us stay on the issue of patriarchy but replace rape culture with, say, dress codes across different countries; there it is much more difficult to say what is acceptable and what is not and even more difficult to judge that one particular practice is unacceptable (say, the burka) while other practices are acceptable (say, school uniforms);
- Alternatively, if we stick to the issue of rape, we can easily see that the clear differences with which we started are, in many ways, historical; so that women used to be punished in Western Europe as well until fairly recently and many would argue that, in subtler ways, they still are punished (see how difficult it is to report rape and especially to achieve convictions).

One can imagine at least two basic approaches to these issues: a *universalist* approach and a *relativist* approach. According to the former—universalism—there is a universally morally acceptable practice and there are universally deplorable practices; and the fact of diversity in both people's beliefs and practices makes no difference to that. According to the latter approach—relativism—there is no universally morally acceptable practices but rather what is morally acceptable is relative to some subset, say a culture, society, community, or something of the like.

Here we should indeed not just distinguish between relativism and universalism but also between two different versions of relativism:

- *Moral* relativism
- *Cultural* relativism

On the one side we have *moral relativism*, which is a meta-ethical theory along the lines of what we have just described: not just the idea that different cultures have different moral practices and beliefs, but the stronger—normative—idea that there is no alternative to such diversity because there are no universally valid moral practices or norms.

Cultural relativism, on the other hand, is a descriptive theory about diversity: it looks at the world and infers from it that there are different moral practices and beliefs—it makes, crucially, no normative conclusion from that diversity; or, better said, one should not take cultural relativism to have normative or meta-ethical implications for the following simple reason: that two people have different views does not show that there is no correct view, as one of them may just be mistaken.

CASE STUDY V: Essen and Berlin

So, for example, my son may think that Essen is the capital of Germany because that is the city where he was born, while I think that Berlin is the capital of Germany. We disagree about the question of which is the capital of Germany and have different views about it; but that does not change the fact that it is Berlin—and not Essen, sorry son—which is the capital of Germany.

When it comes to morals things are quite obviously a lot more difficult than with primary school geography but the point of principle is the same: diversity of opinion does not imply or even suggest that there is no truth of the matter. So—and this is the crucial point for our purposes—*the truth of cultural relativism would neither imply nor suggest the truth of moral relativism.*

A few clarifications are in order: first, as we have just said, the truth of cultural relativism is independent of the truth of moral relativism; it is not just that cultural relativism as a theory may be true without moral relativism being true. The opposite is also the case: moral relativism may be the preferable meta-ethical theory even if there is no actual diversity of morals in the world. This is, again, just because the truth of cultural relativism is an empirical descriptive matter while the truth of moral relativism is a normative issue, albeit a meta-ethical one.

Now that we have distinguished between cultural relativism and moral relativism, let us focus on the latter and no longer concern ourselves with the former. First of all, let me say that, again, the issue of moral relativism is not a purely theoretical one as it has direct consequences on the way we deal with the world around us. It has, for example, an obvious influence on the virtue of tolerance and on what we ought to tolerate as opposed to what we are allowed not to tolerate.

CASE STUDY VI: *The Children Act*

To take a basic case from healthcare, think of Jehovah witnesses who do not accept blood transfusions even in life-saving circumstances (there is a nice novel by Ian McEwan on exactly this topic, *The Children Act*[7]). Are we expected to accept or tolerate that? What room is there to intervene and override their beliefs and preferences? Could we, say, distinguish between adult and children in such a way that we respect adult wishes and not proceed with the transfusion while not respecting children wishes (or their parents') and go ahead with the transfusion?[8]

This is not the place to answer a question as specific as this one (but we will come back to it): it will suffice to notice how the truth of some form of moral relativism is crucial to what we may be allowed to do in such a case of different religious beliefs and practices.[9]

Here is one influential formulation of moral relativism (from Bernard Williams' classic, *Morality*):

> 'right' means (can only be coherently understood as meaning) 'right for a given society' . . . therefore it is wrong for people in one society to condemn, interfere with, etc., the values of another society.[10]

The basic idea has a crucial similarity with noncognitivist views as we have already analysed them: namely, there is a difference in meaning. Just as according to noncognitivists when we say 'torture is wrong' we are really saying that we disapprove of torture, according to the moral relativist when we say that 'torture is wrong' what we are really saying is, as Williams puts it, 'torture is wrong for (my) society'. Relativism, like noncognitivism, restricts the scope of our moral judgements.

There are also crucial differences between relativism and noncognitivism though, which is the reason why we have introduced moral relativism as a sort of compromise position. Moral relativism has more robust truth conditions than noncognitivism, at least if we interpret the statement 'torture is wrong for my society' as something more than just a purely descriptive report on what our society approves of, which then would make it equivalent (if broader) to the noncognitivist 'I disapprove of torture'; for example, 'my society disapproves of torture'.

The alternative would be to interpret the statement 'torture is wrong for my society' as normative, but only within the boundaries of the society where the statement is spoken—so that, within that society, the statement is a norm for all members and not just for the speaker. Interpreting relativism along these lines makes it a more substantial view than basic noncognitivism; still, relativism is subject to obvious objections.

First, because then we would still have to answer the question of where the force of that norm within your society comes from; what's to say that no one within your society could object? So we easily see how the same meta-ethical issues would come back to haunt us. They would be restricted to our society instead of universal but they would be just as challenging—as just replying that the force comes from the fact that society believes x won't do as a normative principle.

Bernard Williams himself points to a much more basic objection:

> [T]he view is clearly inconsistent, since it makes a claim in its third proposition, about what is right and wrong in one's dealings with other societies, which uses a nonrelative sense of 'right' not allowed for in the first proposition.[11]

Williams' criticism is very simple: from the meta-ethical idea that right just means right in a given society, moral relativism wants to derive some sort of principle of universal tolerance—but that's a nonrelativist principle, so one that would be in violation of the whole approach or, at a minimum, that would itself be subject to the basic point that it could only really mean something along the lines of tolerance is right in my society, which would then fall short of delivering universal tolerance.

There are at least two possible replies here: first, the conclusion about tolerance may be inconsistent but that does not say anything about the truth of the first premise, which is alone already a statement of moral relativism. So it may be that we cannot derive tolerance from relativism, but that does not actually falsify relativism understood as the claim that 'right can only ever mean right in a given society'.

A second objection to Williams' critique could be that, actually, we don't need moral relativism to deliver nonrelative tolerance as long as the first premise, which presumably will be true for every society or speaker's context, will each time deliver tolerance for that society. That way we would end up with tolerance everywhere even though we would not have had to appeal to an inconsistent nonrelative conception of tolerance.

Moral relativism, then, is not necessarily inconsistent; but the more important question is: is it plausible? Can it be true? When we look at the rape example with which we started, it certainly seems more than just possible to condemn patriarchal practices, here and abroad: we are actually obliged to do so and to try to change these practices. Here again distinguishing between ontological and epistemological considerations—and also remembering that moral relativism is supposed to be a meta-ethical view rather than a normative one (since it does not commit itself to any actual claims about which actions are right or wrong)—may help us make some progress.

It could for example be that, on the one side, our moral judgements have scope beyond our own society—so that at the meta-ethical level moral relativism would not apply. At the same time, it could be that our arguments for or against practices which are deemed acceptable within other societies or systems need to be much more sensitive to the specificities of such societies. Here it will help to make an analogy with the difference between doing something wrong and being blameworthy for that action.

A person may be in circumstances such that even though he did something wrong we shall not blame him for his action: think of someone in extreme poverty trying to feed his children, for example. We may want to, at the same time, hold on to the moral judgment that, say, stealing is wrong and was wrong even under those circumstances but at the same time we may want to excuse the person in question for stealing, given his particular circumstances. The point is that our judgement should be sensitive to the particular situation which leads to him stealing.

Something similar may be available in the case of relativism: even if moral relativism as a meta-ethical theory should fail, it could be taken to be an important reminder of the difficulties involved in judging people and cultures very different from ours and of the need to study and get to know these peoples and cultures and their practices and values much better before we can judge.

Summary

In this chapter we have analysed the nature of moral questions by first of all distinguishing between descriptive statements and normative statements and showing how ethical statements belong to the latter category. Furthermore, we have distinguished between so-called meta-ethics and normative ethics and have gone on to illustrate different positions within meta-ethics, specifically the broad distinction between meta-ethical cognitivism and meta-ethical noncognitivism, which is crucial to the scope and meaning of ethical statements and therefore, also, to whether they can ever be said to be objectively true. Finally, we have introduced relativism as a further alternative within meta-ethics, and distinguished it from universalism while at the same time also pointing out the difference between moral relativism and cultural relativism.

Notes

1. Just a basic signpost here: I will be using 'moral' and 'ethical' interchangeably throughout.

2. Philosophers often formulate this principle—to go extra safe—in terms of a general principle against "killing innocent children" but I have always wondered about that formulation, as it implies the possibility that children may be something other than innocent, which seems problematic to me.

3. See Jonathan Dancy, 'Ethical Particularism and Morally Relevant Properties',

Mind 92:530–47; *Moral Reasons* (Oxford: Blackwell, 1993); and *Ethics without Principles* (Oxford: Clarendon Press, 2004).

4. This translation is from the Penguin edition of *The Last Days of Socrates*, a book which contains four of Plato's dialogues, all revolving around Socrates' death. The translation was originally by Hugh Tredennick (Harmondsworth: Penguin, 1954), revised by Harold Tarrant (London: Penguin, 1993).

5. Here one could keep exchanging arguments and counterarguments and replies and counter-replies but we don't have time for that. For those interested, a good starting source for further debate on this issue is, like it is often the case, the relevant entry of the *Stanford Encyclopedia of Philosophy*: https://plato.stanford.edu/entries/religion-morality/.

6. The following notorious case provides a chilling illustration of rape legislation and practices in Saudi Arabia: http://www.today.com/id/15836746/ns/today-today_news/t/rape-case-calls-saudi-legal-system-question/#.WOZGc_nygkK.

7. Ian McEwan, *The Children Act* (London: Jonathan Cape, 2014).

8. For example, my understanding is that Danish legislation allows intervention at least in the case of children and override the parents' refusal on 'jus necessitatis' grounds. See: https://www.ncbi.nlm.nih.gov/pubmed/2008754.

9. It should be said that the specific issue of tolerance towards religious belief may be a problem even if we reject moral relativism, as it may be that religious belief deserves special considerations. On this issue, see Brian Leiter, *Why Tolerate Religion?* (Princeton, NJ: Princeton University Press, 2012).

10. Bernard Williams, *Morality* (Cambridge: Cambridge University Press, 1972), 34.

11. Ibid.

CHAPTER THREE

Means and Ends

Kantian Normative Ethics

I would not be at all surprised if the previous chapter had been a disappointment to you: thinking of ethics and right and wrong, you may have been expecting something which would have answered basic questions such as:

- *Should I give all my money to charity?*
- *May I assassinate Donald Trump?*
- *I am pregnant but I don't want the baby: may I get an abortion?*
- *When am I allowed to take a dead patient's organs?*

More generally, questions of the following kind: What should I do? What am I allowed to do? Is doing that my duty? What are my rights?

Isn't giving answers to these questions the point of ethics and moral philosophy? It is, even though, as we have just seen, that's what normative theories do—but there is more to ethics than that and possibly more difficult issues than those ones, as the previous chapter is meant to have shown. Still, answering the question of what we are allowed to do and what we are not allowed to do remains a crucial task of ethics, so this is what we now turn to in this chapter.

The basic ethical question is, you may say, *what shall I do?* Given the tools we have acquired from the previous chapter, we now know how we should understand that 'shall'. It is, namely, a normative 'shall', so that it is not just about deciding in general what to do but it is more precisely about deciding what to do from a moral point of view; to be precise, then, that 'shall' should be more like a 'should' or, even better, an 'ought'.

Already when we try to replace that 'shall' with a more normative term, we encounter the next distinction; namely the one between:

- what we are obliged to do;
- what we are allowed to do; and
- what we are not allowed to do.

Talking of right and wrong is, in this respect, not precise enough, because it leaves no room for the crucial distinction between moral duty and moral permissibility. Still, the idea would be to think of both actions that we are obliged to perform and of actions that we are allowed to perform as 'right' actions, while actions that we are not allowed to perform would count as wrong actions.

This is the basic framework with which we will work, even though we can already see that even this framework has its limitations: not everything that we are allowed to do is, for example, morally good even if it may be 'right' just in the minimal sense of not being wrong. Think of, for example, buying superfluous products or driving when you could have cycled or taken public transport. Of such actions it may be plausible to say that they are 'right' in the basic sense that, since you are allowed to do them, they are not morally wrong. But it's another question whether those actions are good in any substantial sense: as in, do you do any good by performing those actions? Well, to yourself alone, if at all.

Also, this is a good place to clarify that, throughout this chapter, whenever we will be speaking of good, bad, right, wrong, and so on we will always be speaking in ethical (or moral) terms. This is important because there are other contexts to those value-laden words: obviously the legal context, which we have already identified as separate. But also the political context: take the example above of driving when you could have easily cycled.

One option is to say that your driving was, from an ethical point of view, permissible but that there was no good in it—that would be the distinction we have appealed to between 'ethically permissible' and 'ethically good', where the latter implies the former but where there are plenty of cases of the former which do not qualify as ethically good.

An alternative—and this is where the political context comes in—is to say that, actually, for environmental reasons driving when you could just as easily have taken a bike is ethically wrong but that, at the same time, we live in liberal societies where individual freedom, liberty, and state-neutrality are valued so highly that we allow people to do things which are ethically wrong.

Whichever alternative you find more plausible, what's important is to keep those concepts apart: permissible does not necessarily mean good and what is allowed within our political system must not necessarily be thought to be also morally right.

Let us now return to our three 'verdicts', so to speak: obligatory, permissible, and impermissible. Normative ethics can be thought of as the discipline which tries to answer questions about whether some action is obligatory, permissible, or impermissible. It is, in that respect, a very boring endeavour: of any given action, normative ethics is supposed to deliver a verdict. Imagine indefinite long lists of actions, some of which will be deemed obligatory, other permissible, others again impermissible.

Don't worry, though: this chapter will not be made up of long lists of actions and their verdicts. This is for two related reasons: first, what normative ethics is really interested in, more than the actual verdict, is *why* some action is obligatory, permissible, or impermissible. And that—and this is now the second reason—points to some generality: namely, the reasons or justifications why actions are deemed obligatory, permissible, or impermissible need not be as many as the actions in question. Ideally, on the other hand, normative ethics will provide a limited set of principles which can be deployed to work out the moral value of actions. And it is with these principles—and with the different theories putting them forward—that this chapter deals with.

Ethical Egoism

Let us start with a principle which is often referred to as 'ethical egoism' and that is hardly a principle at all—more like anything goes, actually. The crude idea of ethical egoism is that, in its weaker version:

WEAK ETHICAL EGOISM: *everybody is allowed to do whatever they would like to do*; and, in an even stronger version, that:

STRONG ETHICAL EGOISM: *everybody ought to do whatever they would like to do*; so that ethical egoism sounds very much like the *homo homini lupus* of Thomas Hobbes' state of nature: everybody's out for themselves.

This principle—or whatever you want to call it, really—should not be confused with meta-ethical *nihilism* or *amoralism*, according to which there are no moral values: the reason for this is that, however plausible or empty you may take ethical egoism to be, it does formulate a norm, one that nihilists and amoralists would have to reject *qua* norm. On the other hand, though, you could imagine that, at the normative level, ethical egoism would represent pretty well nihilist and amoralist meta-ethical positions.

The other position that ethical egoism must be distinguished from is its psychological counterpart, *psychological egoism*; according to which we can never do anything other than to pursue our own self-interest. With the distinction between descriptive and normative statements now in our conceptual toolkit, we can here use it to distinguish between these two versions of egoism—noting that psychological egoism makes ethical egoism superfluous.

I am not going to look at psychological egoism in any detail here, I just want to note that it is not clear what evidence would count in favour of either its truth or falsity, as psychological egoism would claim, of every action however its content, that the action was done because the agent wanted to perform it. But—and this is the crucial weakness of psychological egoism—that is a pretty empty explanation; and, in the second place, to say that every action was performed because the agent wanted to perform it is not the same as to say that every action is performed in pursuit of the agent's self-interest, for the simple fact that the agent may want to perform an action which is not in her self-interest.

So much on psychological egoism; but is there anything that speaks in favour of ethical egoism? Here, having distinguished between normative ethics and meta-ethics and specifically between ethical egoism at the normative level and amoralism (or nihilism) at the meta-ethical level, it will not do to bring some sort of scepticism about moral objectivity in play to justify ethical egoism; moral objectivity, as we have seen in the previous chapter, remains a big deal in meta-ethics but it cannot be brought to bear twice; so that here the kinds of arguments that will count in favour or against ethical egoism will have to be normative arguments instead of meta-ethical arguments.

One such argument could go something like this: just like conservatives argue that the state should know its limit and leave a lot of regulation to the markets, which will do a better job at it than governments, something along the lines of these kind of market liberalism could be used to argue in favour of ethical egoism. It could go as follows: leave human beings to decide for themselves what is best for them and their fellow human beings and you will see that they will end up coordinating nicely and a lot of good—or not too much bad—will come of it.

Two difficulties here: on the one hand, you may think that the kind of optimism on display above is so crazy that it can only be the result of bad consciousness; so that, really, what is going on in arguing in favour of ethical egoism is the powerful pushing for a theory which will enable them to pursue their ends without any restrictions. This is, after all, the argument for market regulation: in a nutshell, the idea is that without any restrictions whatsoever, markets will not end up coordinating; rather, wealth will be accumulated by increasingly fewer people. The same could be said of ethical egoism: if you don't put any restriction, who is going to protect the few, the weak, the poor?

I am sure the above is no surprise: maybe, I am biased; more likely, ethical egoism is, rather than one possible normative theory within ethics, the rejection of the need for normative theories; and indeed, it may be that there is no need for normative theories; but if there is such a need (if not for everybody, at least for the few, the weak, the poor), then it looks as though that theory will not end up being ethical egoism. So we can move on.

A more substantial variation on ethical egoism could be formulated as follows:

You may do whatever you like as long as you do not harm other people while at it.

This principle has, over ethical egoism, the advantage that it does formulate substantial limits in terms of harming other people being impermissible; at the same time, it shares with ethical egoism that liberal ethos of allowing people to pursue their own conception of the good, as John Rawls would have put it. Here instead of analysing and evaluating the above principle in detail, we introduce what can be considered to be the better known relation of it—Kant's categorical imperative; and while discussing the latter we will contrast it with the above liberal principle.

Categorical Imperative

We now come to what is, arguably, the most famous single principle in the history of moral philosophy: Immanuel Kant's ambition to trace back the whole of ethics to a short formula known as the categorical imperative:

> Act in such a way that you treat humanity, whether in your own person or in the person of any other, never merely as a means to an end, but always at the same time as an end.[1]

This is what is commonly known as the *Humanity Formula* of Kant's categorical imperative.[2] Let us first of all try to understand what the principle says. It is a general norm in two senses: it speaks to everybody—in Kant's terms, every human person anyway; secondly, what it asks of everyone regards everyone else—humanity, or all human persons. Additionally—and controversially—the clause 'whether in your own person or in the person of any other' adds the complication that the principle is not just supposed to find application in everyone's dealings with everyone else but also in everyone's dealings with themselves.

What does the principle ask of everyone with regards to everyone else? To treat them never merely as means but always also as ends. What does that mean? This is complex, so let us start by listing different possibilities that the principle either states or implies:

1. treating someone as a means
2. treating someone as a mere means
3. treating someone as an end

On top of the above three, it will be important to get some clarity on the relationships between those three. From the principle itself it appears relatively clear that Kant takes (2) and (3) to be incompatible with each other and that Kant would at the same time allow for the compatibility between (1) and (3), otherwise why bother with the specification about 'mere' means? But this still does not clarify the important question of whether Kant meant that, as long as we do not treat someone as a mere means, we are treating them as ends; or whether, alternatively, those two really are two different requests upon us, a negative request and a positive request.

The negative request would amount to something that it is impermissible for us to do, namely to treat someone as a mere means; and the positive request would amount to something that it is obligatory for us to do, namely to treat everyone as an end.

CASE STUDY I: *Taxi Driver*

At this point it will be beneficial to introduce some examples. The following case is one I have always thought particularly helpful in this context: imagine taking a taxi to the train station (in fact, when I started using this example, there was no such thing as Uber, but I don't think that it makes any difference; even though Uber's autonomous-cars project may make my example obsolete soon enough). What would Kant's categorical imperative say about your relationship to the taxi driver in the case in which you take a taxi to the train station?

Are you treating the taxi driver as a means? Or even as a mere means? Or are you treating the taxi driver as an end, as requested by the categorical imperative? I think this much is clear: even though, just like in most if not all commercial interactions, you are in a relevant sense 'using' the taxi driver for your purposes, you are not treating him as mere means as long as he is willing to take you to the station (for money, obviously).

Indeed, in the spirit of Uber's dream of symmetrical relationships between service providers and customers, we can see that, here, you are 'using' the taxi driver for your purposes—to get to the train station—just as much as the taxi driver is using you for his purposes—earning money, doing his job, and so on. That is, I guess, the way in which our society works: we cooperate through commercial relationships. In the good cases, everybody's happy: you have been taken to the train station within a reasonable timeframe and have paid a fair price for it, which makes the taxi driver happy as well.

This may admittedly not reflect the reality of social relationships within markets but it does at least help us illustrate Kant's categorical imperative: the difference between treating the taxi driver as a means and treating him as a 'mere' means would then have something to do with the taxi driver's willingness to take you to the station for some X amount of money.

Here it would not be out of the question to combine a bit of Marxism with Kant's categorical imperative in order to argue that, actually, in a lot of cases that have the same structure as our taxi-driver case, we are treating people as mere means—and indeed, whether or not this is fair to Marx, one could even go on to argue that the way work functions within capitalist societies inevitably leads to objectification, namely to the worker being treated as a mere means. This could be, for example, because the worker is not free to reject her wages, as she may not have a decent enough alternative.

CASE STUDY II: *A Textile Factory in Bangladesh*

Think of the kind of textile factories which seem to regularly burn down in Bangladesh—for many workers in these factories, there is not much alternative to a wage cut; they may not be able to get another job and there may not be any unemployment benefits; are those workers mere means within the textile chain? Maybe. But here our focus is not on whether capitalist society is necessarily in violation of Kant's categorical imperative or whether commercial transactions can ever be such that we treat others as means (or even ends) rather than mere means; the point was to distinguish between means and mere means in the first place—and we have done so by appealing to the willing taxi driver, who is not a mere means to your trip to the train station but rather a willing means, just the way in which you are a willing means to his trying to make ends meet and earn a decent wage.

We have distinguished between means and mere means in terms of the other person's willingness to interact with you; and this helps us further, because we can also use it to understand what Kant may have meant with talk of 'ends'—namely, the difference between means and mere means is whether or not the interaction is compatible with the other person's plans or, indeed, ends. With the taxi driver, then, the kind of ride to the train station that you are asking for is the way in which he earns a living, so we can take it to be not just compatible with his ends but actually instrumental to his ends—so that we can say that by taking his taxi to the station we are contributing to the fulfilment of his ends; we are, then, treating him as an end. So our little story would appear to fulfil the requirements of the categorical imperative.

There is a distinction that needs unpacking hidden within our story: on the one hand, one could take it that, as long as the other person is willing, the interaction is instrumental to her ends or, if this other formulation is any help, brings her closer to the fulfilment of her ends. But on the other hand, this does not need to be the case, so that someone may accept an interaction that is compatible with her ends without necessarily being beneficial to her ends. It could be thought that both these alternatives qualify as complying with Kant's requirement not to treat people as mere means but that only one of them complies with the further requirement that we treat them as ends.

The problem is one that we have already encountered: does the fact that we don't treat someone as a mere means necessarily imply that we are treating her as an end or is there room between those two, so that we may not treat someone as a mere means without thereby also treating her as an end, for example—as above—because the interaction is compatible but not beneficial to her ends? After all, people often settle for less than what they would have actually liked.

Here we really have two different questions:

- Does Kant's formulation of the categorical imperative allow logical room between respecting the mere means clause and respecting the ends clause so that we can do the former without doing the latter?
- If there is such logical room, does Kant's categorical imperative actually demand that our interactions with others ought to always be beneficial to them?[3]

This is a big deal and the plausibility of the categorical imperative may depend on which of the two interpretations above is correct. You will recall that we have started from ethical egoism to then move on to a principle according to which you can do anything you like as long as you don't harm others. Now the question is whether we should interpret Kant's categorical imperative in terms similar to that principle—where not treating others as mere means would replace not harming them; so that, as long as one does not treat others as mere means, they are allowed to do what they like. This is, if you like, the *liberal* interpretation of Kant's categorical imperative and can be formulated as follows:

LIBERAL IMPERATIVE: *Do not treat others as mere means.*

As we have just seen, though, this is not the only interpretation available. If there is a difference between not treating others as mere means and treating them as ends; if that difference should be understood in terms of the latter—treating others as ends—but not the former—not treating them as mere means—consisting of only doing things that are beneficial to the other's ends; and, finally, if Kant is asking us to always treat others as ends in the way above, then the categorical imperative looks very different:

SAMARITAN IMPERATIVE: *Always do things that are beneficial to the ends of others.*

It may be objected, here, that the Samaritan interpretation goes too far in the following way: even if we accept all of the above, that still does not mean that we should only do things that are beneficial to the ends of others because the categorical imperative is only about interactions with others so that it can only ask us to further the ends of others when we interact with them rather than all the time.

The point would be that, say, playing videogames or, for that matter, writing philosophy may be legitimate even if it does not further the ends of others for the simple reason that it does not necessarily require an interaction with others. If it did—and all the activities that indeed require interactions—we would be obliged, according to the Samaritan interpretation—to further the ends of others. But as long as we don't interact, that obligation does not apply—and there is nothing in Kant's categorical imperative that obliges us to interact in the first place (at least as long as we don't assume that interaction is a particularly effective way of furthering the ends of others, which it may be).

Accordingly, the Samaritan interpretation of Kant's categorical imperative should be distinguished from other Samaritan views which could be said to be too demanding in requiring us to always do what is beneficial or best for others (we will see later on how utilitarianism may be subject to this kind of challenge).

Even if the Samaritan interpretation can be shown to be less demanding than previously thought, it still raises an important question that we have not yet provided an answer for: namely, whether Kant's categorical imperative should be interpreted as a principle about what we are allowed and not allowed to do or whether it should be interpreted as a principle about what we are obliged to do.

Negative and Positive Rights and Duties

The time has come to introduce two related further distinctions. The first is the distinction between:

1) Negative rights
2) Positive rights

Parallel to this there is the distinction between

3) Negative duties
4) Positive duties

These two distinctions are important in themselves but they will also help us better understand Kant's categorical imperative. Let us start from 'negative duties' as they match well onto something that we are already familiar with, the concept 'impermissible' or 'not allowed'. If I have a negative duty X, that means that X is something I am not allowed to do and that, therefore, X is impermissible.

CASE STUDY III: *'Thou Shalt Not Kill'*

The basic example of negative duty is one that we will discuss in some detail in the chapter after next, namely the commandment 'Thou shalt not kill'. That killing is wrong, not allowed, or impermissible means that I have a moral duty not to kill—and if the principle against killing is meant to be general—namely to apply to everyone—then I have, consequently, a negative duty towards everyone else not to kill them.

This negative duty which I have towards everyone else not to kill them corresponds to a negative right that everyone else has against me not to be killed by me. That's the simple conceptual relationship between negative duties and negative rights: if I have some negative duty X against you, you have the negative right against me that I don't do X to you. Property rights are classic negative rights: your right to the stuff you own can be expressed in terms of a duty, on my part, not to take your stuff.

Negative duties and rights do not exhaust all the duties and rights that we have, though. In many countries, I have the right to healthcare, at least as a citizen. That kind of right, though, is not about things that others cannot do to me. It is, rather, about things that others are obliged to provide me with. So again we have a conceptual relationship between duties and rights, but those duties and rights are different in their content. My positive right to healthcare in Denmark is expressed by the duty of the Danish state to offer me certain services related to medical care broadly construed.

We should not understand positive rights and duties to be necessarily of a social or political nature as opposed to negative rights and duties being of a more personal nature. We have, plausibly, some basic moral rights and duties towards each other independently of the state: it is not just that I am not allowed to break into my neighbour's place, so that my neighbour has, against me, a negative right to her apartment and I have a negative duty not to trespass. We could also suppose that I have positive duties towards my neighbour: for example, the duty to feed her should she be hungry; or the duty to help her children should they be in danger, say.[4]

In more theoretical terms we could say that our social relationships are not constituted just by noninterference principles; they are also made up of help, support, and solidarity. And indeed here we see how crucial the interpretation of Kant's categorical imperative is: should we understand the categorical imperative just in terms of negative rights and duties, or should we rather take Kant to express also positive rights and duties? We now see that this difference is what we were pointing towards in distinguishing between merely *respecting* others' ends and actually *furthering* their ends.

It is not just a question of how to interpret Kant: it is the much broader and more important question of how to understand our personal and social relationships. This question is particularly difficult—but also interesting—because it is at the intersection between ethics and politics. A categorical imperative understood in the simple terms of noninterference—according to which as long as we do not treat others as mere means to our own ends, we are fine—may be more easily defensible than a categorical imperative interpreted in terms of positive duties to further the ends of others. But plausibility or defensibility, here, would come at the cost of reducing the categorical imperative to not much more than the liberal principle of noninterference we derived from ethical egoism, according to which everyone should be free to do what they like as long as they do not harm others.

On the other hand, the alternative interpretation may indeed be too demanding: if we are always meant to further the ends of others, are we ever allowed to look after our own interest? Only, it seems, when our own self-interest happens to further the ends of others—which, in our society, may not be such a rare event, given market forces. So, for example, buying a new car may further our own interest while at the same time furthering the ends of all those who make a profit from it in the commercial chain.

One way of seeing how demanding the categorical imperative would become if we understood it in terms of positive duties is that is not clear what negative rights we would have left. Because obviously, in the case of buying a new car, the difficult question is not whether we are the only ones who profit—as obviously the commercial structure of our society guarantees some distribution—but whether there would have been superior ways of furthering the ends of others than buying a new car. And there probably would have indeed been better ways of helping others with the money that a car costs.

If this is true, though, where does that leave our presumptive negative duty to our property—in this case the money we have, supposedly, earned—if we are not allowed to use it in ways that do not further the ends of others (or, in an even stronger version that we will see is associated with utilitarianism, if we are not allowed to use it in ways that do not maximize universal interests)?

Some limitation to Samaritan principles, then, appears to be not just plausible but also necessary in order not to end up with a near-empty list of negative rights.

Counterexamples to Kant's Categorical Imperative

We have, so far, only discussed different interpretations of Kant's categorical imperative; now that we have analysed different versions and readings, we should turn to whether the principle is justifiable as our fundamental normative guide.

Generality—if we are in the business of looking for a unifying principle—is a virtue of Kant's categorical imperative; but its generality can easily turn out to be a problem if it makes it easy to show why the principle won't do. That is where we will start our assessment. Applying the principle of charity, for present purposes we will disregard the possibility of understanding the principle in its stronger version about furthering the ends of others and restrict our discussion just to the clause about not being allowed to treat others as mere means.

Are we really never allowed—from an ethical point of view—to treat others as mere means? Here Kant's case is complicated by his insistence that it is not enough that we do the right thing: we must *will* the right thing and therefore do the right thing willingly or—which for Kant is the same—freely.

To show how this could be a problem take the taxi driver again: yes, taking us to the train station may be compatible with his ends but do we actually care about that? Indeed, does it even make a difference to us that there is a person driving the taxi? As long as we get to the station on time—our end—do we even care about anything else?

This is again where the market is supposed to come in, as a system which allows the satisfaction of mutually disinterested parties: I don't care about the ends of the taxi driver; the taxi driver does not care about my ends; but the market structures things in such a way that the satisfaction of my goal requires the taxi driver's taking me to the station while at the same time the satisfaction of the taxi driver's goal also requires that he takes me to the station. So it works and everybody's happy even though we don't actually care for each other.

We have already seen the difficulties of the above so we won't get into it again: here the point is just that Kant's moral theory is so demanding that it would not be satisfied with this market solution for mutually disinterested parties; it is not enough that I do not treat others as mere means; I must not want to treat others as mere means.[5]

This issue of whether we should just evaluate motives, actions, or consequences will become particularly relevant when we contrast Kant with utilitarian approaches; for now, we will again apply the principle of charity and put this further complication aside and return to the evaluation of what we have called the *Liberal Imperative*, the idea that we should never treat others as mere means.

CASE STUDY IV: *Taxes and Prisons*

Can it really be that I am never allowed to treat others as mere means? Many cases are indeed sorted out by the distinction between means and mere means, but not all of them. Think of taxes or, alternatively, prison. Nobody goes to prison willingly and most people, if possible, would rather pay fewer taxes. Doesn't that show that our society is constructed around limitations to our freedoms that could be argued to amount to treating others as mere means?

Here we should distinguish the example of taxes from the prison example but they both teach us something important about moral principles such as Kant's categorical imperative. In the case of taxes, we could argue that, in the end, people do consent to the payment of taxes—it's part of the social contract. Whether you agree with this or not, what it shows is the crucial role of consent in determining whether something constitutes treating people as mere means or not.

Prison could also be interpreted as part of the social contract—but it is, actually, more likely brute force. It's not that people consent to going to prison: they are forced; maybe for good reason, but it is a form of coercion. What this shows is that, whatever rights a general principle like the categorical imperative postulates, some actions may result in the forfeiting of some rights. The details of this are important—as being convicted of something criminal does not mean losing all rights within our system, only some—but the basic point is that there is, even within Kant, some scope for doing to people things against their will.

A bigger problem for Kant's categorical imperative is proportionality —it lacks a proportionality condition and that alone, it could be argued, makes it implausible. After all, life is full of compromises; most of the time, we have to choose between two negatives, also when it comes to moral dilemmas. Kant's categorical imperative does not make room for these kinds of ethical compromises, it could be argued.

Think of the difficult decisions and compromises typical to healthcare contexts within limited resources: how are we supposed to choose whom and what to prioritize, according to Kant? Are we not inevitably going to treat the other(s) (namely those left out) as mere means, when we make such calls? Here one could argue that nobody is actually being treated as a mere means, it is just that not everybody can benefit and in the end we must make a difficult decision about who will benefit (say, get the scarce meds) and who will not benefit, but the person who does not get the meds is not a mere means of giving the meds to those who get them.[6]

CASE STUDY V: *Ebola*

There is a more obvious problem for Kant's categorical imperative. Take the case of a dangerous infectious disease (we have recently had the spreading of Ebola, for example). Part of dealing with dangerous infectious diseases will amount to quarantining those who have already been infected to avoid further spreading. It is paramount to the effectiveness of quarantine measures that those who have already been infected be quarantined independently of whether they would like to or not: it is, in short, a form of coercion. Indeed, it's a bit like prison, if you like, with the crucial difference that often those who need to be quarantined have done nothing wrong and, on the other hand, may have been infected as a result of having tried to help contain the infection—think of healthcare professionals in the Ebola crisis.

The kind of coercion involved in quarantine seems to be proportional to the risks involved for the rest of the population, especially if the disease is as dangerous as Ebola. Being deprived of some freedom—when the alternative could be countless more deaths—seems to be a proportional price to pay, whether or not those who have to be coerced are willing to pay it. The problem for the categorical imperative is that the proportionality of this measure is independent from the willingness of those who will be put in quarantine; so that those quarantined—or anyway at least some of them—can be considered to be mere means of the greater aim of avoiding the spreading of the disease.

This, you will agree, is a small price to pay—and one that is ethically justified. But the problem for the categorical imperative is that there is no room for this kind of proportional compromises, where it may be worth sacrificing a minority for the sake of the majority. And the problem is big because there are lots of cases, both historical and hypothetical, that have the structure of a relatively small sacrifice for a larger gain.

This is where Kant's moral theory can be contrasted with what's probably its main rival in normative ethics, so-called *utilitarianism*—which is what we turn to analyse in the next chapter.[7]

There is something that needs to be sorted out first though: you will remember that Kant's 'formula of humanity' of the categorical imperative has that added clause about the principle not just being about how we treat others: the principle is meant to apply to humanity as a whole, yourself included; or, as Kant puts it, 'whether in your own person or in the person of any other'.

How is that supposed to work, given that the principle is about not treating others as mere means and respecting their ends? How can I treat myself as a mere means or, indeed, disrespect my own ends? This is a good place to say something basic about ethics which has not come out yet but that is crucial (and also traceable back to Kant): the so-called *ought implies can* principle. This is the idea that we can only be requested to fulfill moral requirements that it is possible for us to fulfill. If I cannot do something, then I can also not be obliged to do it.

'Ought implies can' is relevant here because one may think that it is just impossible to treat yourself as a mere means or to disrespect your own ends—because that would then have become your new end, so to speak. So, applying 'ought implies can', why would Kant want to ethically prohibit, with his principle, something which is impossible for us to do, namely use ourselves?

Two related points here: first, is it really impossible to use ourselves? Relatedly, Kant may have been trying to anticipate an objection to the categorical imperative by making it applicable to ourselves as well. This is because alongside the kind of objection that we have already seen—namely that there may be times where something is justifiable despite being a case of treating someone else as a mere means—we have the symmetrical opposite objection of some action which may be wrong despite it being compatible with the categorical imperative, so that some action may be wrong even though we don't treat anybody as a mere means.

If the principle is supposed to be basic and generally applicable, this latter objection is just as problematic as the other one; so maybe the added clause about treating yourself as a mere means can be interpreted as anticipating this kind of objection.

Kant does indeed use that clause to condemn things like suicide—where, supposedly, we treat ourselves and our life as a mere means:

> To annihilate the subject of morality in one's person is to root out the existence of morality itself from the world as far as one can, even though morality is an end in itself. Consequently, disposing of oneself as a mere means to some discretionary end is debasing humanity in one's person.[8]

Kantians have also tried to apply the principle in order to, for example, put a moral limit to markets; where despite both parties agreeing to a transaction, we may want to deem that transaction morally problematic.

CASE STUDY VI: From Sex Work to Organ Sales

Take two classic examples: sex work and organ sales. Of both these examples we may want to say, on the one hand, that as long as all parties involved participate freely (namely, as long as the ends and goals of all parties are respected), there is no problem; while, on the other hand, something is still wrong. There may be, in short, wrongs that are beneficial (or at least not harmful) for everybody.

Here the basic Kantian point—in order to argue that those practices can still be wrong even though everybody participates freely in the transaction—is that one does not need to argue that there is objectification between people because there is self-objectification. Namely, we use ourselves as mere means when we sell our organs or sell sexual services.

Still, I don't see how this is supposed to work. Why would the offering—in return for money—of sexual services, as opposed to, say, musical services or educational services, be problematic? If I am objectifying myself if I sleep with a stranger in exchange for money, why am I not objectifying myself when I teach or play for a stranger in exchange for money? Obviously the intimacy of sexual relations makes things more complicated, but it does seem as though applying the categorical imperative to such cases opens up to the intricate issue of starting to distinguish between ends which are legitimate and ends which are not legitimate—why would selling your kidney to feed your children not be legitimate while selling your violin may be permissible?

So this may really be a misapplication of the categorical imperative: still, it was useful to address it not just because Kant may have been himself guilty of this misapplication but also because it has illustrated another kind of argument against the categorical imperative, the idea that there may be actions which are wrong even though they are compatible with the principle.

Having looked at possible problems with the Kantian principle, in the next chapter we will discuss an alternative to it, utilitarianism.

Summary

In this chapter we have finally started trying to provide some answers (well, at least some philosophical answers, which may turn out to be no answer at all for healthcare students and professionals). We have introduced the normative distinction between obligatory, permissible, and impermissible and then looked at some related normative theories, starting from ethical egoism moving on to a basic liberal principle of doing what you like as long as you don't harm others and then comparing that liberal principle with Kant's influential categorical imperative, which we have analysed in some detail, including different interpretations and possible counterexamples. What we have covered is in no way exhaustive, but especially our analysis of the categorical imperative was also meant to provide an exemplary case of how to analyse, criticize, and defend ethical principles.

Notes

1. Immanuel Kant, *The Groundwork of the Metaphysics of Morals*, trans. M. Gregor (Cambridge: Cambridge University Press, [1785] 1996), 4:429.

2. This is, famously, only one formula. The other main formula is the one according to which we should 'act only in accordance with that maxim through which you can at the same time will that it become a universal law' (*The Groundwork of the Metaphysics of Morals*, 4:421). This other formula raises some of the similar questions that we will discuss here, but also some further questions, including the crucial question of what the relationship between the different formula is supposed to be; for example, whether, ultimately,

the different formula are equivalent or at least whether they should be all ultimately reduced to one of them. Those interpretative questions are important—for example, for the issue of the generality of Kant's theory it matters whether it is meant to be reducible to just one principle or whether it actually amounts to a plurality a principle. For simplicity's sake I have chosen to focus on the Humanity Formula here, which is always what I will be referring to when I speak of the categorical imperative without further qualification. For more on other formula and the relationships between them, a good place to start is the entry on Kant's moral philosophy in the *Stanford Encyclopedia of Philosophy*, both the main text and its bibliography: https://plato.stanford.edu/entries/kant-moral/.

3. When we talk of 'beneficial' or 'instrumental' to the ends of others we mean that from our point of view rather than objectively, so *intensionally* rather than *extensionally* (in philosophical speak).

4. Even though, from the point of view of political philosophy, something like this may be the difference between more *communitarian* approaches and republican approaches about nondomination.

5. What that would mean—not wanting to treat others as mere means—is not easily determined. One could think that, given that the taxi driver happens to want to fulfill my goal, in our story I do not want to treat him as a mere means, given the circumstances. But not caring about the ends of the taxi driver could also rather amount to a counterfactual in which getting to the station on time was so important to me that, if the taxi driver does not comply, I am prepared to, say, threaten him with violence. If I am prepared to threaten him with violence, it seems that the bare fact that, as it happens, the taxi driver is indeed willing and there is no need for my threat will not actually be enough in order to say that I do not want to treat him as a mere means. Rather, I am very much prepared to treat him as a mere means but luck has it (or, if you prefer, market forces have it) that I do not need to. I doubt that would satisfy Kant.

6. Here philosophers tend to distinguish between means and side effects but I won't get into any detail here. For more on this issue, see my book *Ethics Without Intention* (London: Bloomsbury, 2014).

7. Here I have admittedly also covered a small fraction of Kant's moral theory. For those who want more, a good place to start is the relevant entry in the *Stanford Encyclopedia of Philosophy*: https://plato.stanford.edu/entries/kant-moral/.

8. Kant, *The Groundwork of the Metaphysics of Morals*, 423.

CHAPTER FOUR

Pain and Pleasure

Utilitarianism and Consequentialism

In its basic version, utilitarianism says that all our actions should maximize utility understood from an impersonal point of view: so not our own utility or that of our family or group; but everyone's aggregated utility—from the impartial point of view of the universe, as it is sometimes said. So in judging an action we should just check whether it has maximized universal utility: if it has, then the action was morally justified; if it has not, then the action was not morally justified.

Let us start from the similarities between utilitarianism and the views we have looked at so far: utilitarianism too appeals to a general principle—sometimes referred to as the *principle of utility*—to which all moral judgements can be traced back to.

The second aspect which utilitarianism has in common with, for example, Kant's moral philosophy, and which on the other hand distinguishes these two from ethical egoism, is impartiality. Utilitarianism—just like Kant's moral philosophy—makes no special case for you, the subject, as deserving any priority—nor does it leave any room for giving priority to, say, your children or your friends.

The impartiality of utilitarianism is, if you like, even more radical: while Kant's moral philosophy may, for example, allow for some benefit for yourself as long as, depending on the interpretation, either—weak version—you don't treat anybody as a mere means or—strong version—you further the ends of others, utilitarianism leaves no such wiggle room. You must further universal utility, stop. From the point of view of universal utility, your worth is just like anyone else's—no special treatment, then.

Utilitarianism is not, in this respect, a *liberal* theory, at least not in the way in which we have been conceiving of liberalism here: there is no space for furthering your interest; all the space is occupied by furthering universal interests. This is somewhat ironic, at least historically, as one of the founders of utilitarianism—John Stuart Mill (together with Jeremy Bentham)—is also one of the principal inspirations of political liberalism.

Partiality

Here it is important to emphasize the *radical* nature of utilitarianism. Taking on the point of view of the universe means that the agent/subject, according to utilitarianism, counts just as much as anybody else. There are two different elements that need emphasizing about the impartial character of utilitarianism. That the utilitarian agent may and indeed ought to only pursue universal interests means both that she may not give any priority to her own interests and that she may not give any priority to the interests of her family, friends, neighbours, countrymen, and so on.

This may appear to be one and the same point but it is actually two different claims, as the comparison with Kant's categorical imperative will help illustrate. This is because Kant's categorical imperative is—no matter how we interpret it—as impartial as utilitarianism when it comes to prioritizing your family, friends, and neighbours over strangers: namely, you may not; everybody's ends should be respected, no matter whose ends they are; just like everyone's preferences and interests count according to utilitarianism, no matter whose interests or preferences these are.

In the other sense of impartiality, though, Kant's categorical imperative may allow for some flexibility that utilitarianism does not allow for: namely, on the interpretation according to which all that is morally required by the formula of humanity of the categorical imperative is not to treat others as mere means, then we may give ourselves some priority, as long as that does not require that we treat others as mere means. So at least the subject or agent—on a particular interpretation of Kant's categorical imperative—may constitute an exception to radical impartiality and may be allowed to be partial to herself and her own ends.

This, importantly, is not an option according to classic utilitarian approaches, where the interests of the agent or subject count, from the point of view of the universe, just as much or as little as the interests of everyone else. In this respect then utilitarianism is even more radically impartial than Kant's categorical imperative. We will see later on in this chapter how this particular aspect is related to the *consequentialist* character of classic utilitarian approaches.

Putting aside for now the interpretation according to which at least the categorical imperative may allow for some partiality towards oneself, what should we make of the radical impartiality put forward by normative theories such as Kant's and utilitarianism? On the one hand, we may admire it: after all, what argument can there be for prioritizing—from a moral point of view—your neighbours over strangers who live further away from you? They too will have ends, aspirations, interests—they too are capable of suffering; they too may have a family. How can we possibly make distinctions based on their location or on whether they are known to us or not? How can these distinctions ever be morally relevant?

This point becomes even more significant once we point out that, indeed, it is often the case that those strangers living far away from us are the ones suffering the most and surely, in most cases, need more help than our neighbours, friends, and family. Here obviously it will not do to appeal to a purely psychological explanation: it may be that the joys and pains of our neighbours are more vivid, just because we can experience them directly, so to speak. But from an ethical point of view, why should that matter? As long as we can know with just as much certainty that far away strangers are suffering—how can we possibly be partial towards those close to us?

This egalitarian and progressive aspect of impartiality is surely something to admire and that we should aspire towards. But there is another aspect to denying people the chance of being partial: namely, meaningful relationships such as those between friends, those between parents and children, those between sisters and brothers, even those between colleagues or neighbours (sometimes), are at least in part the result of partiality. In a completely impartial world, it is not clear that we could maintain such relationships or, at least, it is not clear that these relationships would be as meaningful as they are in our admittedly partial world.[1]

Here it is not just a question of accepting that our world is less than perfect; rather, the point is that a perfectly impartial world may have to pay a price in terms of something that it particularly important to most of us, namely our most meaningful relationships such as those to our children, for example.

On the other hand, if you think of this issue in distributive terms, the following argument may apply: the kinds of harms and benefits which are the result of our world being a partial one are crucial ones because they impact resources such as food or healthcare for people who are extremely poor; while the kinds of harms and benefits which would result from a perfectly impartial world would be of a different value, they would not impact, say, people's survival or basic health needs; it would rather be a question of their quality of life. Put this way, one may argue that the kinds of side effects that may result from a perfectly impartial world may not be compared—in the basic ethical terms of welfare—to the advantages that such a world would have over the partial world we live in.

One final point on partiality: this debate also poses the question of against what we should assess a moral theory or, as in this case, one of its crucial aspects. Sure, obvious candidates are truth and justification, so basically whether there are good reasons, on balance, for some moral theory or moral judgement. But once we look at the further question of what counts as a good reason for some moral theory or moral judgement, two inevitable candidates are plausibility and intuition. Think of all the examples, historical or fictional, that I have been using throughout: in an important sense, what these examples were meant to achieve was appeal to your intuition in order to make some theory or judgement plausible.

Given the normative nature of our reflections, it is difficult to transcend plausibility and intuition; but, on the other hand, when it comes to something as fundamental as the issue of partiality and related questions such as whether we may be partial towards our own children, it is extremely hard to assess those issues in terms of plausibility and intuition; indeed, it could be said that with something like the question of partiality we reach the limits of plausibility and intuition as tests for our moral theories and judgements. Those questions are, if you like, too personal to trust our intuitions; on the other hand, if we cannot trust our intuitions in this case, and therefore we cannot assess the relevant answers in terms of their plausibility, then why should we do that in other cases? And if not on the basis of plausibility and intuition, what else can we appeal to in order to assess those reasons and arguments? Well, as circular as this may sound, the answer may be *reason* itself.

Utilitarianism

Back to utilitarianism: if you combine what we have said about utilitarianism being impartial with its not being a liberal theory, you may conclude that utilitarianism is an *egalitarian* theory. And there certainly is a fundamental sense in which utilitarianism is egalitarian: namely, from the point of view of universal utility, interests are not distinguished accordingly to whose interests they are (indeed, famously Jeremy Bentham was already proposing, in the eighteenth century, something similar to animal rights, arguing that—when it comes to morality—we should not ask whether individuals could think but rather whether they could suffer; thereby extending the moral realm to at least some nonhuman animals).

We should not confuse this impartial idea of the point of view of the universe with the claim that, according to utilitarianism, everyone's interests count the same. Because, in that respect, utilitarianism is more brutal than that: if, for whatever reason, your interests are more relevant to universal utility than your neighbour's, then utilitarianism will prioritize your interests over those of your neighbour. This is the sense in which utilitarianism is not egalitarian: it does not distinguish and discriminate between persons qua persons, but it does allow distinguishing and discriminating between their interests.

An example will help illustrate this point: you and your neighbour are both late for work and you have called a taxi at the same time. Who should take the first taxi to arrive—assuming that there is no way to establish who's taxi that is (again, here Uber may well ruin my examples)? Utilitarianism will just look at what benefits for universal utility there will be from each taking the first taxi—or, and that's the same—what negative consequences could be avoided by each taking the first taxi. Now suppose you are a doctor with a long list of surgeries planned for today and you are already late for your first operation. Your neighbour, on the other hand, works at a call center which is currently trying to sell holiday packages.

This is a case where you may welcome the fact that utilitarianism prioritizes the doctor over the call-center employee: after all, nobody's going to die from not having been offered to buy a holiday package. But egalitarians could not allow for these kinds of prioritizing: it would only further the doctor's privilege. The point here is not whether or not the utilitarian approach is plausible in this particular case (it may very well be); the point is to emphasize the difference between utilitarianism and egalitarian approaches (another obvious example is wealth distribution: if equal wealth turns out not the most conducive form of distribution from the point of view of universal utility, then utilitarianism will not recommend equal wealth).

Already in our discussion of Kantian morality we have encountered both a major advantage and a major drawback of utilitarianism: the major advantage—at least over Kant's moral theory—is that utilitarianism does allow for the kind of moral compromise and proportionality that is shut out from Kantian morality. Taking again the quarantine case: obviously we should put those already infected in quarantine, since that will be best from the point of view of universal utility because we will prevent the disease from spreading.

The point is so obvious that I don't think there is any need to elaborate on it. But before moving on to the already mentioned drawback of utilitarianism, let me point out that the fact that utilitarianism, as a theory, allows for proportionality and compromise may easily be turned against the theory. This is because, from the point of view of universal utility, in order to prevent the spreading of the dangerous infectious disease, a lot of things may be worth doing—a lot of nasty things, like, for example, killing all those already infected if necessary; or, even worse, killing those at most risk of being infected next, just to be sure. If the stakes are high enough, utilitarianism can justify anything: that is, indeed, the whole point of the theory. That may constitute an advantage over Kantian morality in some cases, but it can also be, quite clearly, a big problem. Just look at the scenario below, one of moral philosophy's notorious thought experiments:

CASE STUDY I: *Thomson's Surgeon*

You are to imagine yourself to be a surgeon, a truly great surgeon. Among other things you do, you transplant organs, and you are such a great surgeon that the organs you transplant always take. At the moment you have five patients who need organs. Two need one lung each, two need a kidney each, and the fifth needs a heart. If they do not get those organs today, they will all die; if you find organs for them today, you can transplant the organs and they will all live. But where to find the lungs, the kidneys, and the heart? The time is almost up when a report is brought to you that a young man who has just come into your clinic for his yearly check-up has exactly the right blood-type, and is in excellent health. Lo, you have a possible donor. All you need do is cut him up and distribute his parts among the five who need them. You ask, but he says, 'Sorry. I deeply sympathize, but no'. Would it be morally permissible for you to operate anyway?[2]

Utilitarianism seems to be committed to say, in this scenario, that the surgeon should operate and kill the young man. As fanciful as this little story admittedly is, it makes its point very clear: utilitarianism can justify anything as long as the stakes are high enough. So what started as an advantage over Kant's moral theory increasingly looks like a problem for the utilitarian approach.

This idea that, as long as the stakes are high enough, utilitarianism can justify anything, should not be misunderstood. Here we should distinguish between

- action *types*
- action *tokens*

We can have multiple tokens of a single type, so that the computer I am typing on is a token, among millions, of the type 'computer'; types can be more or less specific, so that we can further specify the type 'computer' by adding that it is a 'laptop computer', that it is an 'Apple laptop computer', that it is a "MacBook Air Apple laptop computer', and so on. Each of these different types will have multiple tokens and each time that we further specify the type, we exclude countless tokens from being tokens of that type.

Having made this distinction, let us now move on to applying it to the claim that utilitarianism can justify anything as long as the stakes are high enough: that claim only refers to action types, not to action tokens. Indeed, utilitarianism will only justify those actions tokens that—depending on the version we embrace—maximize (or at least further) utility. So utilitarianism cannot justify any action tokens but only those that follow the principle of utility.

On the other hand, when we talk of action types, we can see that indeed in principle utilitarianism can justify any action type. Take action types such as cheating, stealing, killing, abusing, and so forth. Each of these types will have tokens that utilitarianism will condemn but also at least possible tokens that utilitarianism will, in principle, have to justify—as long as, indeed, the stakes were high enough for the relevant cheating, stealing, and so forth. Here one could further distinguish between rule-utilitarianism and act-utilitarianism, where only the latter would be subject to this criticism; the more interesting point, though, is about the generality of the theory in comparison with its alternatives—say Kantian morality.

Is generality a good thing for a moral theory? Should we aim for a theory that delivers us general principles against large action types? Not necessarily. After all, the moral theory that we should embrace is the one that condemns all and only wrong actions. On the other hand, if such a theory is not available, then other features of theories will become relevant—and that's where things such as generality and simplicity may come into play—just in the same way in which they may come into play when evaluating scientific theories, by the way.

Now to the (other) drawback: we said, when discussing the categorical imperative, how the idea that one may be obliged to always further the ends of others may be too demanding—philosophers often refer to this kind of Samaritan solidarity as supererogatory rather than something we have the duty to do. We can now see, though, that this is exactly what utilitarianism demands of us: that we always put universal utility first. Indeed, more: that universal utility is all that matters. How can we ever meet the demands of utilitarianism, then?

Here are two possible ways of weakening down utilitarian demands: on the one hand, it could be that furthering universal utility is not a matter of duty; it may be the right thing to do in any given situation without also always being what we are obliged to do. But if we make such a move, it is no longer clear what utilitarianism tells us we should do anymore—we are at a loss as to the basic question 'What should I do'?

An alternative would be to hold onto the obligatory character of the utilitarian demands but to weaken their content by removing the idea that we should always *maximize* utility. Maybe it would be good enough if we always made a positive contribution to universal utility instead of maximizing it: that would still have all the benefits of utilitarianism that we have discussed without being as demanding as the original version.

There are many more things that we could say about utilitarianism; but I cannot hope to do justice to everything here; so I will just mention two final features of it and then move on.[3] Today, within philosophy, people speak of *consequentialism* rather than utilitarianism. So let's clarify what those two concepts stand for: utilitarianism is normally taken to be a consequentialist moral theory. What that means is that the objects of moral evaluation are, solely, consequences; not, for example, motives or intentions; nor whether something was an action or not; just consequences.

When we speak of utilitarianism, then, it would be more precise to speak of utilitarian consequentialism—as consequentialism does not need to be of the utilitarian kind. Indeed, the utilitarian version of egoism—in which all that counts is personal utility—is also best thought of as a consequentialist theory. The consequentialist nature of utilitarianism distinguishes it, for example, from Kant's moral theory where—as we have seen—motives play an important role.

Why is the consequentialist nature of utilitarianism important? We can easily see that if we go back to Thomson's example. There, after all, the problem for utilitarianism seemed to be that the surgeon may be obliged to do—following the principle of utility—something horrible, namely sacrifice an innocent healthy patient to save five sick ones. How could one save utilitarianism from having to draw such a conclusion? One possibility would be to say that, if the surgeon does not intervene, she does not kill the five patients—they die and she could have prevented that; but still, it is not the surgeon who kills them, it is their illnesses.

This reply is a version of what is sometimes referred to as the distinction between killing and letting die or, more generally, the distinction between doing and allowing or actions and omissions. The surgeon does not kill the patients, she merely lets them die—because it is not her doing that kills the patients; it is, at most, her omission that allows them to die. This could be a way for the utilitarian to reject the challenge that the theory is committed to the surgeon killing the innocent healthy patient, at least on the assumption that the difference between killing and letting die is so significant that it overrules the difference between one life and five lives.

Enter the consequentialist nature of utilitarianism: since only consequences matter, all these distinctions above are not open to utilitarian consequentialism, as we should more precisely refer to the theory. When evaluating consequences and consequences alone, it is immaterial whether we talk of killing or letting die, actions or omissions, doing or allowing: it is just the consequences, namely one life as opposed to five lives, that matter.

Here the story could get quickly much more complicated if we introduced such things as, for example, the *Doctrine of Double Effect* or the so-called *Trolley Problem*. But having already written at length on those further issues in my 2014 book *Ethics Without Intention*, I won't get into it here; especially given that the point here was just to explain what it means for utilitarianism to be a consequentialist theory and why this feature is important.

I had promised two features of utilitarianism, so here is the second and last: utilitarianism or, as we have just learned to call it, utilitarian consequentialism is a naturalistic approach to ethics or, at least, it has the potential to be a naturalistic approach to ethics. This goes back to the history of utilitarianism, which started out as a hedonistic approach, namely one which focused on pain and pleasure, so that the basic principle would be about maximizing pleasure and minimizing pain or—taken together—about achieving the best possible balance of pleasure and pain.

It is easy to see the naturalistic promise of such an approach if we think of it in meta-ethical terms instead of purely normative terms: if the question is the grounding of ethics in nature or, at least, in objective facts, the focus on pain and pleasure promises to deliver that by making two measurable variables the crucial variables of ethics: at least in principle, the balance of pain and pleasure is something which can be measured. It is, therefore, something that we can judge empirically and objectively. Hedonistic utilitarianism would then answer the big unanswered question of ethical objectivity by reducing ethics to pain and pleasure.

More than that, actually: focusing on pain and pleasure has the further advantage of choosing concepts over which people have clear attitudes: pain is bad, pleasure is good. So this approach promises both objectivity and a simple answer to the why question. But obviously things are not that simple: reducing morality to pleasure and pain is like making the following equations:

pleasure = good = right
pain = bad = wrong

Those equations will, themselves, have to be justified; and this is not just because people may happen to like pain and dislike pleasure. Moreover, these equations, if left unanswered, would amount to what philosophers call the *naturalistic fallacy*: the idea that something is wrong because it causes pain derives something normative (X is wrong) from something descriptive (X causes pain). But this clearly does not follow: we need the extra premise—and that's crucially a normative premise—that pain is wrong. Deriving (X is wrong) directly from (X causes pain) without the added normative premise that (pain is wrong) would be an example of committing the naturalistic fallacy—and that's bad.

But if the reason why pain should be minimized is that pain is wrong, then utilitarianism no longer has an account of 'wrongness', for which instead it would be appealing to some independent standard. This problem should not come as a surprise: in discussing meta-ethics, we warned against achieving objectivity through naturalism at the cost of making ethics contingent. We have now encountered an example of just that worry.

There is another problem with hedonistic utilitarianism, one that the early utilitarians had already recognized. Take John Stuart Mill's famous remark:

> It is better to be a human being dissatisfied than a pig satisfied; better to be Socrates dissatisfied than a fool satisfied. And if the fool, or the pig, are a different opinion, it is because they only know their own side of the question.[4]

This remark points to the evolution of utilitarianism from Bentham's hedonist version which focused on pain and pleasure—remember the point about asking whether a being can suffer rather than whether it can think—to Mill and his distinction between higher and lower pleasures, which is much closer to today's talk of satisfying preferences and interests.

Here the point is not Mill's controversial prioritizing of the educated over the uneducated or of human animals over nonhuman animals; rather, the interesting aspect of leaving pure hedonism behind is that focusing on preferences and interests allows much more flexibility for the principle of utility: after all, our life is much more complicated than just pleasure and pain. Still, there is a price to pay with this move from hedonism to higher pleasures: namely, the naturalistic aspect of utilitarianism is gone and with it its promise of measurability and empirical objectivity. But as we have already seen that such promise might have been illusory anyway, maybe this is a price worth paying for utilitarians.

There is one final aspect of the comparison between utilitarian approaches and Kantian approaches that we should mention and that speaks in favour of the former over the latter: questions of distribution, which are particularly relevant within the healthcare context. Sometimes doing the right thing is a question of knowing how to distribute scarce resources: we are very familiar with this issue when it comes to the distribution of wealth and issues of wealth inequality.

Just as there can be *wealth* inequality and just and unjust distributions of wealth, there can also be *health* inequality and just and unjust distributions of health or, more appropriately, healthcare. Indeed, healthcare as a whole could be considered to be a scarce resource that we must distribute justly. More commonly, academics and policy makers debate, for example, distributive questions when it comes to such scarce resources as organs (think of *triage*). Everyday around the world people die who are waiting for an organ transplant: organs are a paradigmatic example of scarce resource.

Here I don't want to get into the debate about the distribution of scarce resources within healthcare, just point to the difference between Kantian and utilitarian approaches when it comes to this particular question. It is easy to see how utilitarian consequentialists will deal with such questions: they will evaluate the consequences of the different distributive models and argue in favour of the distributive model which is preferable in terms of universal utility. There may be cases where two models are equal in terms of universal utility—as the case of two patients, each waiting for an organ, where there is no utility-based reason to favour either. But, in general, a principle of utility will mostly be in a position to choose between distributive models.

It is more difficult to see how Kantian approaches would choose between distributive models: remember, the starting premise is that the relevant health resource—say organs—is scarce, which means that demand is higher than supply. How are we then supposed to choose between competing interests, in such cases, by applying the categorical imperative? By definition, all parties want or are interested in or have the end of obtaining the resources in question; also by definition, we cannot satisfy each party—with scarce health resources, indeed, equal distributions are more difficult because you can't very well split a kidney in two and give each half a kidney.

So the categorical imperative alone does not give us a distributive principle, apart from whatever we can derive from the idea that we should not treat others as mere means—but that alone does not tell us who we should give the one kidney to—and apart from the idea that we should respect—and maybe even further—the ends of others, which would suggest that we should, when possible, give both parties a kidney, shame we just have one kidney to transplant.

Summing up, when it comes to distributive questions utilitarians seem to have an advantage: utilitarianism may sometimes get stuck when it comes to distributive questions, but Kantians get stuck all the time. Here is where we could introduce, for example, John Rawls's veil of ignorance to put forward alternative fair and just distributions—but that's beyond the scope here; all I wanted to do was further illustrate the differences between the two approaches by appealing to the question of the just distribution of scarce resources.[5]

From Theory to Practice

Our answers over the last two chapters have been so general that I fear hardly any disappointment will have dissipated. On the other hand, we cannot provide an answer to each of the moral dilemmas that people face; and not even to the majority of moral dilemmas that healthcare professionals alone face. What we can do, though, is to apply the principles that we have analysed in the last two chapters to provide some exemplary answers, which will contribute both to further clarify the principles and the differences between them and also may provide some guidance as to how to answer all the other questions.

What I will do is take the four practical questions that I put forward at the beginning of chapter 3 and try to give a reasoned answer to each of them. Here are those four questions again:

- *Should I give all my money to charity?*
- *May I assassinate Donald Trump?*
- *I am pregnant but I don't want the baby: may I get an abortion?*
- *When am I allowed to take a dead patient's organs?*

Before I start, let me clarify that I am not claiming that ethics has to be able to provide an answer to these or other particular questions; it could be that all ethics can provide us with are conceptual tools rather than answers, which would then be the responsibility of individuals. But, as we said early on, ethics is a practical endeavour; so it will have to at least be able to provide possible answers to practical questions.

CASE STUDY II: Should I Give All My Money to Charity?

Should you give all your money to charity? I genuinely don't know. On the one hand, we have seen how utilitarianism—with its principle about maximizing utility—may oblige us to do all we can in order to at least improve universal utility. Whether, on the other hand, giving all your money to charity is the most effective way to make a contribution to universal utility is mostly an empirical question which will depend on your circumstances, your talents, your future; so, for example, it may be that, on your deathbed, the best you can do for universal utility will indeed be to donate all you own to charity—instead of giving it to your children, for example; which does say something substantial about the justification of the practice of inheritances.

But if you still have many working years ahead of you, it may be that the best way to contribute to universal utility is a breakthrough within your field, for example (that will admittedly hardly ever apply to philosophers; but it may be more relevant to those working within healthcare—on this, see the so-called *effective altruism* movement).

So whether people should donate all their money to charity is a question that will also depend on their factual circumstances. But the question has a possibly more important aspect to it over which we may be able to say something substantial: namely, the fact that most of us are partial in our preferences and behaviour; partial towards family and friends, for example; partial towards people of our own nationality, race, or religion; but also partial towards the welfare of people near us—who we can see, hear, whose pain we can feel and empathize with; as opposed to people who are different from us; unknown to us; far away from us.

As we have already discussed, it is very difficult to see how the theories that we have looked at within the last two chapters could possibly justify this form of partiality towards those close to us—in this respect, whatever their differences, theories such as Kantian morality and utilitarianism share a fundamental impartiality from which we can take inspiration.[6]

CASE STUDY III: May I Assassinate Donald Trump?

The question is somewhat provocative, especially as it involves a living person. But the point behind it is an important one: the value and justification of political violence. Assuming a rejection of total pacifism and strict nonviolence—even just on the grounds that some self-defence is certainly justified or that war may sometimes be just—we are faced with the difficult question of the morality of violence towards those that have the power to affect the lives and welfare of millions of people.

On this point we have a clear difference between Kantian morality and utilitarianism, at least when taking both in their brute form. On the one hand, Kant makes no exceptions for members of humanity based on their conduct—everybody is and remains a human being; that is, after all, also the point of *human rights*, that they are supposed to be no-matter-what rights. Utilitarianism, on the other hand, has the tools to justify political violence, as long as the powerful are powerful enough, you may say. But it obviously makes a difference whether or not the powerful in question can be claimed to be rightful representatives of their people, as the result of fair elections, for example.

So the answer to our question is probably no; but the reason for such a negative answer is possibly not that it is never legitimate to exercise political violence; the reason may rather have to do with Trump's procedural legitimacy.

CASE STUDY IV: I Am Pregnant but I Don't Want the Baby: May I Get an Abortion?

This is one of the classics in bioethics. Abortion—also because of religious stances on it—has been at the forefront of both academic and public debates around bioethics. It is customary to talk—at least for the political debate—of prolife and prochoice stances, where the former identify those who argue that it is prima facie wrong to abort and that this should be prohibited (maybe with the exception of extreme circumstances such as rape); prochoice defenders of abortion will usually argue that it is a question of the woman's autonomy so that abortions may be justifiable independently of the status of the foetus (for example independently of whether it should be considered to be a person or not—this is the position that, within philosophy, has been famously defended by Judith Thomson in *A Defense of Abortion*).

For Kantian morality the abortion issue is particularly difficult because, if the foetus should indeed be considered to be a member of humanity, then killing it—whatever the benefits for the mother—will be treating the foetus as a mere means, thereby violating the categorical imperative. On the other hand, it will be difficult to convincingly argue that a foetus, at any stage of development, should be given full membership of the community of persons (even though we should not confuse this last point with the idea that at every single stage before delivery the organism should still count as a foetus, a further issue which is relevant to the ethics of late-term abortions, for example).

Additionally, as we have mentioned, the fact that the foetus is either a part of the woman's body or at least *within* the woman's body makes the issue one of bodily and personal sovereignty—one in which moral norms against abortion are, ipso facto, also norms that interfere with women's bodies. This, rather than the metaphysics of personhood, seems to be the most convincing argument for the permissibility of abortion—especially given the problems with a strict interpretation of Kant's mere means prohibition that we have already identified within the last chapter.[7]

CASE STUDY V: *When Am I Allowed to Take a Dead Patient's Organs?*

Here I will say very little since a lot of the relevant issues turn on death and consent, which happen to be the central issues of the next two chapters. But the basic idea is that through organ transplants we can save lives at a minimum cost, as the organs come from the dead. What is taken to be crucial, within the bioethical debate, is that the dead have somehow consented to donating their organs. It would be at least in theory possible to argue that organs could be taken independently of the wishes of the person who has just died, but not many people go that far, even though the utilitarian argument for this conclusion appears to be pretty straightforward.

What's particularly interesting here, from the point of view of Kantian morality, is whether even dead persons could count in terms of infringements on the categorical imperative; and indeed if we assume some form of consent is needed, what we are saying is, in a way, that if we don't previously obtain consent, we are treating the dead person or her body as a mere means to the end of saving someone else. And it is certainly not obvious that the dead should count at all in this respect.

Once some consent requirement has been granted, the issue normally turns on how strong such requirements should be; whether for example an opt-out system of organ donation—where people are taken to have consented to organ donation as long as they have not explicitly dissented—would be enough to satisfy consent requirements. Here an interesting issue is whether the state should be allowed to somehow coerce or anyway pressure its citizens to think about something as personal as their own forthcoming death. It would not be unreasonable, it seems to me, for a citizen to object to this aspect rather than to object to donating organs itself; but then probably an opt-out system would be an effective way to also deal with this problem about the state's interference with personal matters: people would end up donating their organs once they are dead without necessarily having had to deal with the issue when alive.[8]

Summary

In this chapter we have introduced a further ethical theory, utilitarianism or, as we have learned to more precisely refer to it, utilitarian consequentialism, according to which actions ought to maximize universal utility and should be judged solely based on their consequences. We have analysed some crucial aspects of this theory (for example, its impartial character and the difference with egalitarianism), emphasizing both similarities and differences from the Kantian morality of chapter 3, such as utilitarianism's aspiration to be a naturalistic ethical theory. We have concluded the chapter by asking and trying to answer four practical ethical questions as a way of testing the theories that we have learned about so far in the book.

Notes

1. On the topic of partiality, see Simon Keller's 2013 book of the same title, *Partiality* (Princeton, NJ: Princeton University Press).
2. J. J. Thomson, 'The Trolley Problem', *The Yale Law Journal* 94, no. 6 (1985): 1395.
3. As always, a good place to start for further readings are the *Stanford Encyclopedia of Philosophy*'s relevant entries and bibliographies. For example the following two: https://plato.stanford.edu/entries/utilitarianism-history/ and https://plato.stanford.edu/entries/consequentialism/.
4. John Stuart Mill, *Utilitarianism* (London: Parker, Son, and Bourn, 1863).
5. On Rawls, see his classic *A Theory of Justice* (Cambridge, MA: Harvard University Press, 1971) and also the relevant entries in the *Stanford Encyclopedia of Philosophy*: https://plato.stanford.edu/entries/rawls/ and https://plato.stanford.edu/entries/original-position/.
6. On the issue of charity and partiality, a classic philosophical read is Peter Singer, 'Famine Affluence and Morality', *Philosophy and Public Affairs* 1, no. 3 (Spring, 1972): 229–43 (available at: http://www.jstor.org/stable/2265052).
7. On the issue of abortion from a philosophical point of view, I recommend reading Judith Thomson's *A Defense of Abortion Philosophy and Public Affairs* 1, no. 1 (1971): 47–66 (available at: http://www.jstor.org/stable/2265091) and Don Marquis's *Why Abortion Is Immoral The Journal of Philosophy* 86, no. 4 (1989): 183–202 (available at: http://www.jstor.org/stable/2026961).
8. On the issue of organ donation, I can recommend Cecile Fabre's *Whose Body Is It Anyway?* (Oxford: Oxford University Press, 2006).

CHAPTER FIVE

Life and Death

The Ethics of Dying in Healthcare

What's the point of medicine and healthcare? It would not be implausible to answer this question by simply saying that the point of medicine and healthcare is to prevent and delay death. And already here we encounter some difficulties: first of all, what does it even mean that the point of medicine and healthcare is to prevent death? Death cannot be ultimately prevented; we are all going to die in the end—so, really, we are left with delaying and pushing back death as much as possible as the more likely aim of medicine and healthcare.

Even this more modest aim of delaying death is not obvious, though: and to see that, we should first of all point out that even if we agreed that delaying death was the primary aim of medicine, it could hardly be the only one; indeed, part of what we aim at in curing disease does not have to do with preventing or delaying death but rather with preventing, eradicating, or lowering pain and other disfunctions—and those do not necessarily have to be related to premature death.

The Aims of Healthcare

Broadly construed, we could say that the aim of medicine and healthcare is to prevent and cure disease (where that includes pain and malfunction, more later) and to prevent and delay death—and that these two aims can be related but need not be. We may prevent or delay death by preventing or curing disease but that is not always the case.

There are at least two kinds of cases where, indeed, the two come apart in important ways:

- Sometimes delaying death may not be conducive to alleviating pain or malfunction—indeed, sometimes alleviating pain may require giving up the other aim of preventing or delaying death;
- Other times we may, in order to cure, bring death forward—as in cases in which a risky operation may have great benefits but may also cause the patient's death.

We have so far identified two basic aims of medicine and healthcare:

- Preventing and delaying death; and
- Preventing and curing disease and pain.

These aims can go hand in hand but they are also often not related to each other and, more problematically for our purposes, they can also be incompatible with each other as in the two scenarios that we have just illustrated. One radical possibility, in order to avoid those difficulties, would be to stipulate that the aims of medicine and healthcare should be restricted to preventing and curing disease and pain without also including preventing and delaying death, which could be considered an upshot of preventing and curing disease.

This suggestion would solve the incompatibilities above—but would it still express the basic reason why we care about medicine and healthcare so much? Fear of death, to put it very crudely. The incommensurability of our mortality and the constant awareness of it, after all, transcend disease and pain: as in, eliminating disease and pain makes no difference to our mortality even though it will, in at least some cases (well, very many, actually) delay death. So the problem is that death—especially our own mortality—is really at the centre of our valuing medicine and healthcare but that, at the same time, making death prevention as the primary aim of healthcare runs us into all sorts of difficulties, including with relation to the other stated aim of preventing and curing disease.

At this stage you may wonder why we are defining medicine and healthcare in such negative terms: isn't there a more positive outlook available? One possibility would be to think of healthcare not in terms of what it wants to prevent, cure, eliminate, or delay (disease and death) but rather in terms of the positive outcomes that it wants to bring about: making sick people

more in general this applies to its potential impact on any normative question) would similarly be guilty of a sort of naturalistic fallacy of deriving a normative conclusion about the permissibility of assisted suicide from a nonnormative premise about the aims of healthcare.

The crucial question here is whether establishing the aims of healthcare is a normative endeavour. If it is not, then either it cannot have normative consequences or there must be some further normative premise that has to be made explicit. Here I am afraid that we need to introduce a further distinction that has been implicit in our discussion so far but that's too central to leave unexplained: the moral (or ethical) does not exhaust the normative, because there are norms which are not moral norms. We should still think of the moral as an example—maybe the primary one—of the normative but start to think of the normative as a larger domain of which the moral is one, albeit significant, component. The implication of this is just that if something is not a moral or ethical issue that does not mean that there is no normativity involved at all.

CASE STUDY II: *Your Colleague's Wallet*

Good examples of this are the norms of rationality. Take the following example: suppose you haven't got any money on you to buy lunch (which, these days, probably mostly means that you haven't got either cards or phone with you, rather than cash—or, worse, your back account is actually empty). You notice that your colleague next door has left her old-fashioned wallet on her desk when going to a meeting and you can see that her wallet has actual banknotes in it. As you have no reservation against stealing money from your colleagues and you believe that your colleague's money will more than cover your lunch, you 'borrow' the necessary amount and go buy your lunch.

There are two different kinds of normativity (at least two anyway) involved here: there is the basic ethical norm that stealing money from your colleagues is wrong, which puts you under *moral* normative pressure not to steal from your colleague's wallet. But there is also a possibly more subtle normativity involved. Given your desires and beliefs (you want lunch; you haven't got any money on you; you see money which would cover it on your colleague's desk; you don't believe that there is anything wrong in taking it), you are also under *rational* normative pressure to steal your colleague's money, because that is an effective way of fulfilling your aim to buy lunch.

This little story shows that normativity is not just moral normativity; there is, for example, rational normativity. So, going back to our question of the aims of healthcare, we have the following three possibilities (at least):

- The question of what the aims of medicine and healthcare are is itself an ethical question;
- The question of what the aims of medicine and healthcare are is not itself an ethical question but it is still normative in some other way;
- The question of what the aims of medicine and healthcare are is an empirical (or at least descriptive) question.

Like in the previous chapter, then, the question is not just what the aims of healthcare are but more crucially what is their status. Basically: who decides what the aims of healthcare are supposed to be? The answer is, at first glance, disappointingly simple: society does, we do, collectively. But at the same time, democratic decision-making processes are not themselves above ethical scrutiny, so that in the end even though the norms that regulate the aims of healthcare are not themselves ethical norms, they must be consistent with basic ethical principles.

The Ethics of Dying

And that's where it all comes back to the ethics of dying. The first thing we should make clear about the ethics of dying is that it is obviously a topic which transcends medicine and healthcare and can be traced back at least to the basic principle against killing which is, for example, one of the traditional Judaeo-Christian commandments: 'Thou shalt not kill'. So that's the default from which debates start. At the same time, in the particular context of medicine and healthcare, this default also corresponds with an ethos of saving life and curing disease, as we have seen throughout this chapter.

This is how we could put things in very rough terms: there is a basic principle against killing which applies to every person; on top of that, within healthcare there is a life-saving ethos which, if you like, is specific of healthcare. Think of the classic 'Is there a doctor on board?': it is not implausible to think that healthcare professionals are subject to some kind of higher standard, given their skills (more on this in chapter 8).

Combining this basic principle against killing and the life-saving ethos of healthcare gives us a preliminary idea of just how controversial the issue of euthanasia and assisted suicide is within medicine and healthcare—and that's before one adds extra complications such as the horrible history of euthanasia within Nazi Germany, for example. In a nutshell: how could we ever expect doctors, of all people, to kill—once we have added the medical ethos to a basic principle against killing?

CASE STUDY III: Killing Is Wrong, Isn't It?

Let us start from the beginning though: namely, from a general principle against killing which we shall preliminarily formulate in terms of 'killing is wrong' which is, really, the equivalent of the commandment 'Thou shalt not kill'. What we want to know is, in the first place, if the principle according to which 'killing is wrong' is true or justifiable.

We will clearly need a lot more detail than this general 'killing is wrong'; while, for now, there is no need to further analyse the predicate 'wrong'—which we will keep taking at face value as we have done so far—there are at least three other variables which need making more precise within 'killing is wrong':

- whose killing is being evaluated by the principle?
- Should we understand the verb 'to kill' as expressing an intentional action?
- Is the principle meant in general terms—as in, 'killing is always wrong'?

Each of the three questions above offers a way to make the principle more specific and, supposedly, also more plausible. Let us start from the first question: if we limit the principle to the killing of human persons by human persons, we may rule out already a lot of difficulties that may have to do with, say:

- (nonhuman) animals killing (nonhuman) animals;
- (nonhuman) animals killing human(s) (animals); and
- human(s) (animals) killing (nonhuman) animals.

All three of the above are complicated and controversial in different ways and make the evaluation of our basic principle against killing even more intricate so we are, for simplicity's sake, going to rule them all out and understand the principle as one referring, solely, to human animals killing human animals—indeed, even more narrowly, to human persons killing human persons; to also rule out, say, cases of killing by small children (other controversial cases such as mental disability or neurodegenerative disease are, on the other hand, relevant for the euthanasia debate so that it would be unhelpful to rule them out at the outset).

A first specification of 'killing is wrong' is then that 'killing of human persons by human persons is wrong'. The second question is meant to rule out accidents and unintentional actions such as mistakes. Take the following case: sometimes human persons kill other human persons as a result of an accident or by mistake, maybe because, on a stage, a gun which was supposed to be unloaded was actually loaded, unbeknownst to the actor who is supposed to pull the trigger.

CASE STUDY IV: *Never Events*

Within healthcare tragic mistakes also happen—in medication dosage, for example; or during operations. Think of so-called *never events*: the US Department of Health estimates that more than 70 percent of never events are fatal and that, in the United States alone, every year more than four thousand *surgical* never events occur (and surgical never events are just one of many types of fatal mistakes).[1] We are therefore easily talking of thousands of deaths every year in the United States alone as a result of never events.

We could have a complex conceptual dispute about whether these events should count as killing events as opposed to accidental deaths, and which of these killings should count as intentional killings, and further which of these, whether accidental or unintentional, are such that someone is morally responsible for them. Each of these distinctions is complex and important, but it is beyond the scope here (but see chapter 8 for more details on questions of responsibility): the basic point is just that not all deaths are intentional killings, not even all deaths caused by human persons.

Again, for simplicity's sake we shall restrict our principle against killing further to only include 'intentional killing of a human person(s) by (an)other human person(s)' (the plural is just there to remind us that we are not necessarily talking in singular terms, neither for the perpetrator nor the victim).

Before moving on to the third question, let us take stock: we have so far narrowed down the basic 'killing is wrong' to 'intentional killing of human persons by human persons is wrong'. The final question is possibly the most complicated: is it always wrong?

One could imagine that the original commandment was either meant as a general principle meant to say that 'intentional killing of human persons by human persons is always wrong' or, alternatively, that 'intentional killing of human persons by human persons is prima facie wrong'. The former version means that, no matter the circumstances, if an action counts as 'intentional killing of . . .', then that action is wrong. The latter version allows for extreme circumstances where an action may be justified even if it counts as 'intentional killing of . . .' but it holds on to the idea that the basic fact that the action is one of 'intentional killing of . . .' will count against it from an ethical point of view; it's just that in this latter case there may be outweighing circumstances.

We have made some progress in specifying the basic principle against killing but before we can apply it to the ethics of dying within healthcare, we need to answer the other obvious question: why is 'intentional killing of human persons by human persons always/prima facie wrong'? The interesting feature of this further question is that it is a legitimate one to ask even if one were to disagree with both the idea that killing is always wrong and with the idea that killing is prima facie wrong. One would, then, just ask the following question: when killing is wrong, why is it wrong?

The Wrongness of Killing

A first simple way in which killing could be said to be wrong is the following: everybody is afraid of dying, nobody wants to die, and so killing someone would disrespect that person's wish not to die. This is a plausible account of the wrongness of killing, if a bit of a superficial one; nobody likes parking tickets either, but giving a fine is not as bad as killing. This analogy may seem a bit funny, but it is meant to emphasize that if the wrongness of killing entirely depends on being killed violating a preference against dying, then the wrongness of killing is just like any other preference violation—which, most people will want to say, it is not; killing is much worse than violating people's preferences in other ways.

There is a simple way out of this problem, though: we can just think of the preference against dying as being not just one of many preferences but rather a crucial defining preference which we value more than most other preferences. Not all preferences are equal just because we value and disvalue things differently—normally, say, your preference against dropping your iPhone on the ground will be valued less (by both yourself and others) than your preference against being run over by a car (even though, who knows with kids today and their iPhones). So the idea would be that, say, there may be circumstances under which people will be willing to violate your preference against dropping your iPhone—either for your sake, their sake, or other people's sake. So if you have to be rushed into an ambulance after an accident, both yourself and others may be willing to take the risk of dropping your iPhone, for example.

The simple point, then, is that the wrongness of killing would not just depend on the violation of some preference: it would depend on the violation of a deep-rooted preference which, for most people most of the time, is one of the things that they care about the most. And yet even this very simple point is already opening up other potential problems with the wrongness of killing: what if people do not have a preference against dying? Or what if people have some preference against dying but they do not rate it as highly as one may expect and, indeed, have things that they care more about?

This issue could be sorted out relatively quickly if, say, everybody always cared about their own survival more than they cared about anything else in the world (there would still be, mind you, other issues with the wrongness of killing, but at least the present problem would be put aside). But we don't live in such a world: people care a lot about their own survival, but they would not always rate it as their first priority. And even then, it is their survival that they care about, not necessarily the survival of other people, known or unknown. So even that may not be enough to show that killing is always wrong.

The problems with the wrongness of killing are, actually, even more basic: first, that someone does not want something to be done to them does not mean that it is wrong to do to them the thing they don't want. Again, who likes taxes, parking tickets, traffic, prison, being turned down for a job, and so on? So the simple fact of not wanting something is far from enough to make the thing in question wrong.

Additionally, we have the issue that we have already seen about people having different preferences and also rating their preferences differently. Then again, if we give up on the idea that killing is always or prima facie wrong, and if on top of this we also give up on the idea that, when killing is wrong, it is always wrong for the same reason, then the above difficulties may no longer be much of a problem.

Nobody thinks that killing is always wrong anyway—well, we could have a long theological dispute about whether the commandments should be interpreted that way, but at least since Aquinas it is pretty clear that even theologians accept that some killing may be justifiable—famously, in Aquinas's case, self-defence.

And you don't need to be Thomas Aquinas to come up with plausible cases in which killing is not wrong. The more difficult question is what happens when we accept that killing is not always wrong. That is, after all, the point of general principles: they are easy. Good to memorize, simple principles such as 'thou shalt not kill' provide guidance even if they are not infallible; which suggests that they may have their merit even if they turn out—as in this case—to be false or at least implausible.

Side note: one may think that I am proceeding too quickly in dismissing the plausibility of the general principle 'killing is wrong'. After all, we had distinguished between the idea that 'killing is always wrong' and the idea that 'killing is prima facie wrong' and while cases such as just war, self-defence, and so forth may provide good arguments against 'killing is always wrong', those arguments do not necessarily transfer over to 'killing is prima facie wrong'.

This is a fair point but it really opens up the question of how we should interpret 'prima facie wrongness': if it is just meant as 'killing is almost always wrong' or 'killing is always wrong expect in extreme circumstances such as . . .', then the point is trivial and we still have to do the work of properly distinguishing between the cases when it is and the cases when it is not—so, really, we have not salvaged very much of the generality of the principle; it would just be a case of what we said earlier about fallible general principles still being pretty useful.

There is an alternative though: namely, the idea that 'prima facie wrongness' is not a question of whether or not we allow for exceptions but rather a question of killing always counting against the justification of a certain action; so that we would say that, sometimes, an action which involves killing may still be overall justifiable but the fact that it involves a killing will always count against it—it would always be a negative, so to speak. This is, indeed, a more promising interpretation of 'prima facie wrongness' but I wonder whether it does work in the case of killing: if some bastard is coming for your children, killing that person is—it seems to me—going to count in favour of the action being justified. It is not a question of lesser evil or collateral damage; so that it's not just that killing is sometimes necessary, it is rather that it is sometimes morally right or, even, obligatory. Similar points can be made about the killing of particularly horrendous or dangerous individuals.

Assisted Suicide

So it seems that killing is not always wrong. How does this conclusion help us with the difficult cases that we encounter within healthcare? It doesn't, actually. Had we been able to look at euthanasia, assisted suicide, and end-of-life care through the lenses of a solid general principle against killing, things would have been easy—maybe not fair, but at least easy from a theoretical point of view.

Here we should make two preliminary distinctions: first of all, it is not only within healthcare that we find this extremely difficult case of someone who wants to die. We are obviously thinking of suicide, which is an issue that transcends healthcare.

The second distinction has to do with something that we have already emphasized, namely the life-saving ethos within healthcare. This is important because it could be used to argue that, even though killing is not always wrong in general, it is always wrong within healthcare. 'Do no harm' is, after all, one of the basic principles of the healthcare professions (more on this in the next chapter).

But, as we have seen, a lot turns on what constitutes harm and, more generally, we cannot just derive what is ethically allowed and what is not ethically allowed within healthcare from the basic aims of healthcare—ethics has, as we have argued, priority here. So that we will have to do ourselves the work of finding out what is permissible and what is not when it comes to end-of-life care.

We could formulate the basic question in the following terms: is a doctor or other healthcare professional ever allowed—from an ethical point of view—to help a patient die, or even kill the patient?

Two aspects of this basic question need clarifying here: as we have seen in the previous chapter, here one must distinguish between the question of what healthcare professionals in end-of-life care are allowed to do and what they may be—always from an ethical point of view—obliged to do. After all, the default is that patients are entitled to healthcare and that healthcare professionals are obliged—within professional limits—to provide care. So what here the basic distinction between duties and permissibility points to is the big issue of whether dying is part of the healthcare provision that patients are entitled to.

The second aspect is that, clearly, there are very many different ways in which this awful dilemma can present itself and talking in general of assisted suicide and euthanasia does not really do justice to the variety of circumstances within end-of-life care. Below are some variables that are particularly relevant for the purpose of ethical assessment:

1. there are patients who are terminally ill and patients who are not;
2. there are patients who are in great pain and patients who are not;
3. there are patients who are conscious and patients who are not;
4. there are patients whose immediate survival depends on the support of some automated system and patients who can, say, breath unaided and feed themselves.

Each of the above brings its own complications but we can say at least the following: (1) may be relevant because one could speak of accelerating death rather than causing death—as in, the patient would have died anyway and the doctor, in the relevant case, would have just provided assistance with other elements which are also crucial to healthcare: whether the patient died after great suffering or not, for example; or whether the patient died in a heavy-on-machinery intensive care unit instead of a more comfortable bed, or even at home.

Those are not, mind you, arguments in favour of euthanasia—they are, much more modestly, just supposed to provide elements that everyone in the debate will agree are relevant from the point of view of the patient's welfare and, therefore, from an ethical point of view. Whether any of these elements make any difference to the ultimate moral judgment over a particular case or principle is, then, a different question.

Point (3) is crucial, on the other hand, because it makes a difference in terms of the patient's wishes. It would be easy—for argument's sake—to just restrict our discussion to cases where the patient wishes to die; but point (3) reminds us that even this move is not that obvious in the context of assisted suicide and euthanasia.

From a purely theoretical standpoint we can clearly just stipulate that the only cases we will deal with are cases where the patient wishes to die. But what does that mean? Take the following scenario: a patient is in a vegetative state and the family finds a diary entry from years earlier which can be quite conclusively interpreted as indicating that, at the time of writing, the patient expressed the opinion that she would not like to be kept alive in a nonreversible vegetative state.

Does that mean that the patient, who is now—let's assume—in a non-reversible vegetative state, now wishes to die? Can we infer from a diary entry about a possible future state a current wish? On the other hand, nothing stops us from again stipulating that all these cases are also themselves too difficult and that we shall restrict our assessment to cases where the patient can now express the wish to die.

A note of caution here: the benefits of argumentative clarity will almost always have to be balanced against possible losses in terms of plausibility or relevance, as for example in the case in which we rule out a great number of relevant cases because they are too difficult to analyse for our theory. Sure, delimiting the scope of our investigation is legitimate; but it must not take place at the cost of relevance; in a slogan: the difficult cases must be dealt with too rather than just left on the sidelines by a neat theory.

There is also another problem with the stipulation that we shall restrict our ethical analysis of assisted suicide and euthanasia to cases where the patient can now communicate the wish to die. Namely, it is not obvious that the fact that the patient can now communicate the wish to die should be given priority, in terms of how we regard the patient's wish, over a case in which the patient previously wrote down hypothetical wishes. What reasons do we have to take actual current wishes more seriously than hypothetical past wishes?

The most liberal approach may here also be the easiest: namely to acknowledge all wishes and to weigh each of them equally, whether or not it is current, communicated, or hypothetical. This does not solve all problems—as there will be cases in which there are contrasting wishes, either across time or, say, between the family and the patient's past wish. Still, it gives us a platform to include not just current communicated wishes but also those of patients who are no longer enable to express them.

We don't need to answer the question of why patients' wishes should be taken into consideration—the answer is obvious: it's their life. But we still need to answer the related question of whether patients' wishes should be regarded as sufficient (rather than just necessary, otherwise it's probably murder). Given that it is indeed, after all, the patient's life that we are talking about, maybe there is a more plausible way to ask the question: rather than why the patient's wishes should be sufficient, what could speak against just going along with the patient's wishes? This is the question that we now turn to.

The first thing we should say on whether the patient's wishes should be enough is banal: dying is a big deal; it is, for example, irreversible. There is no coming back, which is why we don't want to get it wrong and we want to be absolutely sure. This is not something peculiar of dying: irreversible changes—becoming a parent, for example—are commonly taken to be particularly important decisions exactly because of their irreversible character.

This is not a trivial matter, as it could be taken to be grounds for having a kind of life-default, according to which, say, we take it that nobody wants to die if not otherwise stated; or, even more importantly for our purposes, we could take it that a death-decision must have higher standards—for example higher epistemic standards—than other decisions.

Take the following example: it is sometimes said that, before marrying or some other important commitment, one should be sure; and contrast this with buying a new bicycle or settling on where to go out for dinner, where one wants to get it right but does not care that much about making a poor choice. Along these lines, it could be easy to imagine that, when it comes to the decision to die, epistemic standards are even higher.

We may ask what it would be for epistemic standards to be higher or lower: how much do you need to have thought about it? How much information do you need to have consulted? How many alternatives should have been presented to you? Those are important questions, but a more poignant one is: why should death be subject to higher standards?

This question gets even trickier once we include the other ways in which the decision to die may be different: not just epistemic standards may be higher; it could be proposed that, more in general, standards of justification should be higher when it comes to death. Namely, your wish to die will only be taken into account when there is a serious and proper reason for it. What could that be? Well, illness, for example; or pain that cannot be alleviated.

But who should decide that, say, a loss in the family is not a good enough reason? Who would dare making such calls? We see then that this issue of which standards should apply to the decision to die is very complex. And that is why defaults matter: namely, the above is often used as a reason to argue against assisted suicide and euthanasia on the ground that, exactly because it is so hard to make such difficult calls as the ones above, we should never be asked to make such calls; and therefore we should not even allow for the possibility of euthanasia or assisted suicide—because we don't even want to get into the business of making such distinctions when it comes to dying, and the very possibility of assisted suicide and euthanasia would put both doctors and patients in this impossible position (David Velleman, for example, is an influential philosopher who argues along these lines—see his *Against the Right to Die*[2]).

Why should death receive the above special treatment, though? Why not trust people with their judgment and wishes even when it comes to the most fundamental decisions? Indeed, isn't it exactly when it comes to those life choices that we should regard it as most important to respect people's autonomy?

What do I have, after all, from a free society which trusts me enough to choose among different products but does not allow me to choose whether to die and how to do so? Isn't on the latter kinds of choices that we should measure whether or not a society is free? Whether or not the government trusts their citizens' judgement?

Suicide and Assisted Suicide

In at least one important respect, the above is too quick: namely, we should distinguish between suicide outside the healthcare system and euthanasia and assisted suicide within the healthcare system; the latter is the more intricate topic and it won't do to deal with it by using arguments that may only apply to the former, after all.

How could we justify allowing for suicide but not allowing for assisted dying within healthcare? First, one could just argue that all suicides should be prevented; but, as long as one is willing to concede that at least some decisions to commit suicide must be respected, that opens us the difficulty of squaring that with a total ban on assisted suicide within healthcare. And still, restricting such a total ban to healthcare could be justified in at least two ways:

- the life-saving ethos within medicine and healthcare (as we have already discussed this, I will not look at this possibility any further);
- the fact that, when it comes to assisted suicide, doctors and other healthcare professionals are asked for their support.

This latter consideration could be considered to be crucial, so that the difference between suicide and euthanasia would not have anything to do with medicine and healthcare as such but rather with the doctor or other healthcare professional's involvement.

The basic idea is the following: we respect people's wishes to die but are not willing to support those within healthcare. There is, after all, a basic difference between committing suicide and asking someone else to kill you or to help you die. But I wonder how much weight we should give to that difference. If we acknowledge a patient's wish to die so that we would not interfere were the patient to be able to kill herself, shouldn't we offer our support if the patient is not able to do it alone? After all, the reason why the patient will not be able to kill herself without our support will in most cases be a medical one; so that one could even go as far as claiming that the kind of support involved in assisted suicide is part of the care that healthcare professionals owe to patients.

It is in the nature of philosophical questions that one could go on forever, but I think our discussion so far should suffice as a rough guide to the ethical issues around the end of life. Before concluding, just one note of caution: we should distinguish between ethical arguments in favour of assisted suicide and calls to legalize (or, indeed, prohibit) some such practices, as there is a gap between the two; since it may be plausibly argued that such matters are better left to the judgement of individual doctors and patients rather than legislators and administrators.

Summary

This chapter discussed what is probably the hardest topic, both within healthcare and beyond: death. Specifically, we addressed the question of whether healthcare professionals are ever allowed to kill a patients or at least assist them in killing themselves. We have explained why this question is particularly difficult within the context of healthcare (basically, the life-saving ethos within medicine); at the same time, we have looked at the similarities and differences between our increasingly liberal attitude towards suicide outside of healthcare and persisting prohibitions against assisted suicide within healthcare. Is there a tension between these two and if so, how can it be resolved? Answers are particularly difficult in this context but, basically, if we should ever respect a person's wish to die, it is not clear why this attitude should stop at the gates of the hospital.

Notes

1. For more data and information, see: https://psnet.ahrq.gov/primers/primer/3/never-events.
2. D. Velleman, *Beyond Price: Essays on Birth and Death* (Cambridge: OpenBook Publishers, 2015).

CHAPTER SIX

Yes and No

Consent and Paternalism

The topic of this chapter—consent—is one that has already come up in most of the previous chapters, so that we are already somewhat familiar with both the concept itself and also its importance. And indeed, consent is one of the basic principles not just of bioethics and medical ethics but, more in general, of our social life.

To get us started, here are two classic definitions of consent:

> *In the relevant sense, consent transactions have a distinct structure: agent A consents to B's f-ing on A, under a certain description of f-ing, whether or not the offer was initiated by B. For example, a man may consent to a physician's touching the man's testicles as part of a testicular cancer exam.*[1]

> *[consent makes it] 'permissible for A to act with respect to B in a way that would be impermissible absent valid consent'.*[2]

It makes sense to work with both these definitions because they focus on two distinct aspects of consent: the former focuses on what consent is—the structure of consent transactions—while the latter focuses on the kind of normative power that consent possesses: namely, consent can turn otherwise impermissible actions into permissible actions.

The normative power of consent goes even further, actually: an action that would be impermissible given the absence of consent may, once consent has been obtained, become not just permissible but obligatory. Take the case of a healthcare professional, for example, who will be obliged to provide care rather than just permitted to do so, but only on the (crucial) condition that consent has been granted.

Our discussion of consent in this chapter will follow exactly the above double-structure, focusing both on what consent *is* and on what consent *can*: those two questions are, in fact, related but distinct. What we need to find out, basically, is, in the first place, under what conditions it can be legitimately said that someone has consented to something; and, secondly, in which cases consent has this peculiar power of transforming impermissible actions into permissible (or even obligatory) ones—the question is, if you like, what are both the foundations and also the limits of consent's power.

What Is Consent?

The simplest case of consent is perhaps one that has the following structure: two equals agree on a course of action.

CASE STUDY I: *Coffee Break*

Imagine asking your colleague if she wants to take a coffee break or asking your wife if she wants to have lunch together or asking your friend if she wants to go out for a beer this evening. Already these very basic cases have some interesting features: first of all, those are cases of joint action, so that the person doing the asking doesn't just need permission; she actually needs cooperation, *voluntary* cooperation.

This points to a first important distinction: there are cases in which we ask someone else whether he agrees to X where X is a joint endeavour, while there are cases in which we ask someone else whether he agrees to X where X is not a joint endeavour but still we need permission from the other person. So, as opposed to having coffee, beer or lunch together, think of the doctor asking the patient whether he consents to his testicles being inspected; think of asking your colleague whether you can borrow her bicycle; think of asking a stranger on a train or café whether he minds you sitting next to him.

These latter cases are different from the original ones in that the agent could, in theory, just go ahead and do the thing in question, thereby coercing the other party to his testicle being touched, her bike being taken, the seat next to him being occupied by a stranger.

Here are two further features of these cases that we may note: first, that in between these cases there may be ones of which it is more difficult to say whether they belong to the joint action group or whether they are more a case of asking for permission: sex, for example.

CASE STUDY II: *Sexual Relations*

Sexual relations are so intimate and at the same time so diverse that we may both classify them within the joint action category—towards which I would personally rather tend—or within the basic permission category.

I mention the example of sexual relations to emphasize the following point: it is not as if the former joint action cases should be understood as lesser cases of consent; what's crucial to the consent requirement is the potential violation that fulfilling the consent requirement avoids; and in some cases of joint action—as for example sex—the violation is clearly more important, both to the agent and in general, than in, say, the case of borrowing a bike or sitting next to a stranger.

The other element worth reflecting upon is the difference between asking someone whether you can do something to them and asking someone whether you can take or use something of theirs; so for example the testicle case as opposed to the case of borrowing someone's bike. Still, those two cases have something in common: the person whose consent is needed has some authority—maybe even a right—such that not obtaining that person's consent would be a violation of that authority or right; and this applies both to our property—such as a bike—and to our body, which is *ours* in a different way.

Those are, as we have anticipated, the easy cases. They are easy in the following way: they are mostly cases in which both parties are, more or less, equal. In this respect they should be distinguished from the original case of the doctor asking a patient whether she can inspect his testicles. There you may think that there is a significant asymmetry, one of both knowledge and power—one, in a word, of authority broadly understood.

Something along those lines could be said of someone asking an employee instead of a colleague out; saying no or dissent, given a certain power structure or asymmetry, may be more difficult or anyway have a different meaning. Even the case of husband and wife, within a patriarchal society, may be easily constructed in terms of a power asymmetry. These asymmetries are important because, in cases which are particularly serious, they may invalidate consent altogether (you may be familiar with the feminist slogan 'all sex is rape'; that's an example of the above where the context is supposed to invalidate consent altogether; as in, given a certain context, there are no conditions under which consent will count as legitimate; slavery is probably another example of this). And this shows that consent has to be, in some relevant sense, *voluntary*.

Another way in which our cases are easy is that they are constituted by questions and answers, while often consent does not function in terms of questions and answers. Indeed, think of the case of asking a stranger on a train whether he minds you taking the seat next to him: probably in such a case most people, if no reaction at all came, would assume that the stranger did not mind; they would not ask again, or formulate the question in a different language or more loudly, for example. They would simply take the seat.

It is interesting to ask why people would take the absence of some form of dissent, in the above case, for permission to take the seat. I think there are two different elements at play here: on the one hand, an empty seat next to you on a train does not belong to you in any formal sense (apart from the extreme case in which you have bought two different seats not to be disturbed, maybe). So that, normally, it is really just a form of courtesy that we ask whether we may occupy the seat; we are, really, entitled to a nonreserved empty seat on a train or in a café.

Something different may be at play here though; namely the idea, already encountered, that sitting next to a stranger in public would not be much of a violation of that person's privacy, intimacy, or personal space. It would not, in short, be a serious issue, and this lowers the consent requirement so that the absence of dissent may be enough. So here we have two independent difficulties: on the one hand, consent transactions do not just happen along the clear lines of, say, private property and bodily integrity; they also happen along a continuum of more difficult cases where sensitivities may reasonably differ. On top of this first difficulty there is the fact that some potential violations would be more serious than others.

What this great diversity points to is the following: there will be cases where we need legislation to precisely individuate under what conditions consent will be valid; and there will be cases where, even though legislation may not be the appropriate solution, it is important to establish the conditions for valid consent; further there will be cases in which—either because of the complexity of the situation or because the case may just not be serious enough—diverging practices may be acceptable.

Healthcare cases are, within the above spectrum, some of the moral delicate cases: first of all, because many healthcare cases will have to do with bodily intimacy. Secondly, because many healthcare cases will also involve some asymmetry between the parties, as with the case of a doctor, being the expert with knowledge and power, and a patient, who in the majority of cases will have both less knowledge and less power than the doctor. A third element makes healthcare cases particularly important: the stakes will often be very high. Summarizing:

- bodily intimacy
- power asymmetry
- high stakes

Those three elements don't just add up: they multiply, so that bodily intimacy will be felt even more strongly when the stakes are high, for example—and the same goes for power asymmetries.

This may explain why—when talking of healthcare—we often don't just generally talk of consent but rather of *informed consent*. This points to a second necessary condition on valid consent: consent, in order to be valid, must not only be voluntary but also informed—the former is, if you like, an ontological condition while the latter is an epistemological one. Even though we will see in a moment that the ontological condition is really a normative one.

It is easy to see why both conditions are necessary: if someone threatens you with a knife in order to steal your phone and you agree to give him your phone to avoid him cutting you, then you have not consented to him taking your phone. He has rather coerced you into giving him your phone. And this is the case even though you did have more than one option: you could have given him your phone—as you did—or you could have resisted at the risk of being cut. A threat, in short, invalidates consent.

A threat invalidates consent because it fails to meet the voluntariness condition: if you are under threat, your consent is not voluntary; it is, therefore, not valid consent. But there are subtler ways of getting what you want without coercion. Imagine a doctor who really wants a patient to agree to an operation—maybe because the doctor, paternalistically, knows that the operation will be the best option for this patient; or maybe, more egotistically, because the doctor hopes that performing this particular operation will advance her career.

One way for the doctor to make sure that the patient will agree to this operation will be, for example, to downplay the risks: this may be achieved by failing to mention some particular risks or side effects; or by choosing to mention those studies which have shown lower risks or fewer side effects instead of other studies which have shown higher risks or worse side effects; even more subtly, the doctor may choose to use certain more positive adjectives, or a more persuasive tone; or, worse, the doctor may put pressure on the patient or use terminology that the patient will struggle to understand so that the patient will hardly have the courage to ask follow-up questions.

These are just a few examples of the many ways (or tricks?) in which someone in a position of authority and, further, with the epistemic privilege of her particular skills and knowledge can persuade another person to agree to her preferred course of action. Looking at these examples, it is clear that the basic case of coercion is not enough to capture all the different ways in which we can fail to obtain valid consent. If a doctor, for example, knowingly withholds from a patient relevant information about possible risks, then the patient's consent will have been invalidated. And in this latter case—crucially—the condition that the consent transaction will have failed to fulfil will not be the voluntariness condition but rather the epistemic condition which requires that consent be—as it has now become common to say—*informed*.

You may think that there is another side to the epistemic asymmetry between healthcare professionals and patients: namely, that there is a reason—a good reason—for the asymmetry. We want difficult medical decisions to be taken by experts; that is why doctors and other healthcare professionals are educated and trained: to put them in a position to make the right call and execute it accordingly.

The asymmetry, in short, is a good thing or, at least, it is the result of the useful practice of distribution of labour. Which raises the question: why invest so much in healthcare and in the expertise of doctors and other medical professionals if, then, we are not going to trust them with difficult decisions?

Isn't informed consent in healthcare getting things backwards by asking patients to participate in decisions over matters that they cannot understand? In a slogan: Let the experts decide! I think that this is a problematic simplification but that the issue does raise an important question which we must address.

First the simplification: patients are not being asked to make medical decisions; rather, their permission is being asked about the implementation of a medical decision which has been taken by an expert; and their permission is being asked for good reason, as the medical decision will have, first and foremost, consequences for the patient.

The case of risk will help us illustrate this point: the *evaluation* about risk values and probabilities will be made by an expert on the basis of evidence; indeed, most patients would probably not be in a position to make such evaluation. But it is ultimately the patient who will be *taking* the relevant risk.

CASE STUDY III: *That 10 Percent Chance*

Take the following case: your doctor tells you that undergoing a certain operation has 90 percent probability of resolving your health problem and 10 percent probability of causing complications which are worse than the problem you currently have and could possibly even be fatal. This is very broad but will do for our purposes, as it helps us clarify that there are two importantly different senses of evaluating risk; it is the doctor's job to, on the basis of evidence, give an expert opinion of relevant risks and their probability. In this respect, healthcare professionals evaluate risks.

But there is a different sense of risk evaluation which is really up to the patient: namely, to decide if it is worth it. Because the kinds of considerations that come into this second sense of risk evaluation are not medical ones: they are personal considerations about quality of life, for example. Does your health problem currently impact your quality of life to such an extent—or can it be expected to do so in the near future—that you are willing to take a 10 percent risk of dying in order to resolve your problem? This is not a question that a doctor can answer: and that's not just because they may lack some personal information about your private life. It is because it's really up to you to decide *what* is important to you and *how* important it is.

There is a more basic question that still needs answering though: namely, what's the point of consent? Why is it so important? The answer to this question is one which we should really already know: autonomy. It is, after all, our life and our body. Think again of the risk-assessment case: who else is supposed to decide whether a certain quality of life improvement (say, being able to walk again) is worth risking one's life for? Who else is supposed to decide whether a 10 percent or 20 percent risk of fatality is worth it if the alternative is never walking again?

CASE STUDY IV: *Hip Replacement*

Take the following example: hip replacement surgery, especially with patients who are old and may have other conditions, may be necessary in order to be able to walk again but can also have serious consequences; for example, in terms of infections resulting from surgery that older patients already suffering from other conditions may not be able to fight—especially given the vicious regress of antibiotics.

Who else should decide whether to undergo such an operation if not the patient (or, maybe, her family)? It is indeed a very difficult decision to have to take, but no one else can take it if not the patient and her family.

Here one could object that consent is only superficially a way for the healthcare system to respect the autonomy and wishes of patients. What is actually going on—it could be argued—is that the healthcare system is outsourcing critical decisions—and, crucially, responsibility—onto patients, who often don't have enough information or experience to make the right call.

Two different points here: on the one hand, this talk of 'making the right call' is misguided as, in some cases, there may not be a 'right' call: reasonable people may disagree over whether being able to walk again is worth a 20 percent fatality risk; and they may disagree not just because it is difficult to work out, as it may also depend on one's life expectancy, for example; rather, reasonable disagreement will also be due to different people having different preferences—walking is a pretty basic function and it will have different meaning to different people.

Still, even if there was such a thing as a 'right' call in some of these extremely difficult situations, it seems that it is only the patient or her representatives that can be in a position to make that call—with the obvious added difficulty that, once we are talking about the patient's representatives instead of an autonomous agent herself, then there is a genuine question as to whether they may have better access to the patient's preferences than healthcare staff.

Independently of talk of 'making the right call', there is also a question of responsibility here. Consent practices could indeed be seen as ways of avoiding having to make difficult decisions on the part of healthcare professionals while, at the same time, one fails to assume responsibility for what may happen, because the patient had been informed of the relevant risks.

Having patients make the difficult decisions might indeed be an easy way out for healthcare professionals, but that does not mean that it is wrong—again, it's the patient's life and her body that we are talking about. What this rather shows, I think, is the paramount importance of putting the patient in the position of making the best possible decision for herself; again, informing the patient is the best way of empowering her to do what's best for her.

Still, I can't help but suspect that at least some of the informed consent requirements and related bureaucracy of recent decades do fit in rather well with the move in the commercial sector towards offloading as much work as possible onto the customer. We may call it participation and inclusion but it is also, in the end, more work for customers and less work for companies. In this respect it is important to establish when consent requirements are necessary as opposed to cases where we can trust healthcare professionals all the way.

Part of establishing the scope of consent is also finding out how far consent can go. Go back to our original distinction between cases in which the consent transaction works in the permission form—A asking B whether A can do or take something which involves B or belongs to B—and cases where consent is to joint action, as having lunch together. The latter, you may have suspected then, are not cases of consent at all; or, anyway, they are not relevant to the healthcare context, where it's always of case of healthcare professionals asking patients whether they may do something to them or with their property—specifically, within healthcare, that property will often be sensitive information or data.

It is not as simple as that, though: the difficult cases that we have analysed in the last chapter, after all, are cases where the patient asks the doctor to do something to them or to help them do something together—namely euthanasia and assisted suicide. Can consent go that far? We have analysed this question and its possible answers in detail in the chapter on life and death so we will not go into it again here; the point is just to emphasize the difference between the basic question of when consent is necessary and the rather more complicated question of what consent may be sufficient for.

CASE STUDY V: *Clinical Trials*

Clinical trials may be another relevant example here: it is not just a question of consent being necessary in order to involve a patient in a trial; imagine the clinical trial involves a patient who is in critical condition and who wants more meds or a higher dosage because he hopes this will help him (or maybe it's a question of earning as much as possible from the trial). These are also cases where, in one sense, it is up to the agent—if he is the only one to bear the risk.

What this points to is the idea that once we have recognized respect for autonomy as the reason behind consent requirements, then we don't just have the question of when consent is necessary but also the question of what consent is sufficient for: isn't the only true respect of the patient's autonomy not just to respect his wishes by not interfering with them but also to respect them by helping patients fulfil them?

This is, again, the basic distinction between negative duties and positive duties; and we have already recognized that healthcare professionals will have positive duties—basically the duty of care—towards patients. But this makes it difficult to establish a boundary for such positive duties, especially when a needy patient asks for help in the form of extra therapy or, even, assisted suicide.

Paternalism

This brings us to what is, traditionally, the other challenge to consent requirements in healthcare: paternalism. Namely, sometimes respecting the patient's wishes will mean that the patient will be, at least from an external medical point of view, worse off. So that healthcare professionals may want to paternalistically override the patient's wishes—for the sake of the patient herself, that is.

Here are two case studies about paternalism which I borrowed from Bette-Jane Crigger's *Cases in Bioethics*[3]:

CASE STUDY VI: Joe

1. Joe, eighteen years old and unmarried, sustained a severe spinal cord injury in a motor vehicle accident. His arms and legs were paralyzed. He initially required mechanical ventilation, and later a tracheostomy. Three months after his injury Joe was transferred to a spinal cord unit several states away for his rehabilitative care . . . Several nights after placement of the button,[4] the resident on call was summoned to evaluate Joe for respiratory distress. His respiratory rate had increased and his blood gas indicated mild hypoxemia. He was having a great deal of difficulty managing his secretions, despite one-on-one attention from the staff for cough assistance and oral suctioning. The resident on call felt that the tracheostomy tube should be replaced immediately, but Joe refused. 'I'd rather die than have that replaced', he said. The resident explained to him that it would be a temporary measure to insure clearance of secretions and appropriate oxygenation. Joe remained adamant.[5]

CASE STUDY VII: Ms W.

2. Ms W. is a nineteen-year-old unmarried woman pregnant for the third time, having previously had an abortion when fifteen, and a daughter now ten months old. She was admitted to the hospital in the twenty-sixth or twenty-seventh week of gestation and placed on intravenous medications (magnesium sulfate) to stop preterm labor. Two days later, Ms W. asked her physician, Dr C., to discontinue the medications because she was 'tired of being in the hospital and the medications and the fetus were too painful and uncomfortable'. Dr C. explained that the potential risks of premature delivery include: respiratory immaturity, intraventricular haemorrhage, neurologic handicaps, and even fetal death. He advised her to continue the medications for two to three more weeks to give the fetus more time to mature. These critical weeks would enhance the fetus's chances of survival (from 50 percent at twenty-six weeks' gestation to 90 percent at thirty weeks' gestation) and decrease morbidity, reducing the risk of chronic lung disease (from 50 percent at twenty-six weeks' gestation to 20 percent at thirty weeks' gestation) and neurological handicaps later on in life. Ms W. continued to refuse treatment . . . Dr C. contemplates three options: Respect Ms W.'s wishes and risk delivering a very premature fetus who may expire or may survive and be handicapped secondary to prematurity and its complications; refuse to abide by her wishes,

but transfer care to a physician who is willing to do so; refuse to abide by her wishes and try to obtain a court order to force Ms W. to undergo treatment.[6]

Those two cases share the following structure: the patient has some wish X which the doctor thinks is not in the best interest of the patient (and, in the latter case, we may also add that the doctor may think the patient's wish is also not in the best interest of the foetus). This is, if you like, the other side of consent: in both cases, the doctor needs the patient's consent in order to be able to proceed with treatment; otherwise treatment would be, at least prima facie, impermissible. So such cases of paternalism raise the important question of whether consent is always necessary or whether sometimes healthcare professionals may be allowed to start or continue treatment even without the patient's consent.

It is worth emphasizing that both cases above are a particular kind of lack of consent: namely, the patient is explicitly asking for treatment to be discontinued. As in, both patients are actively communicating their wishes and making them very clear to the doctor. This is important just in case someone thought that there was a relevant ethical difference between lack of consent and explicit dissent, where the latter is a subset of the former, but somehow stronger: if there were such a difference, these cases should certainly count as explicit dissent rather than mere lack of consent. Both patients are saying, loud and clear, no to treatment.

There are good utilitarian reasons for continuing with treatment: the patient in the first case study, Joe, will probably die if the tube is not replaced or anyway have further dangerous complications; one can understand the patient's frustration and fear—even panic, maybe—and still replacing the tube is a relatively minor procedure given what is at stake. In the other case there seems to be even stronger reasons that speak against interrupting treatment given the chances that the foetus will develop all sorts of problems if it is delivered too early.

This latter case is admittedly complicated by the whole abortion issue, but that does not make too much of a difference in the end: if the patient was asking for an abortion would be one thing but the patient appears to prefer early delivery, which would have disastrous consequences for not just the foetus but also the mother, given that her life would become much more difficult and complicated with a disabled child, for example.

In a certain way, then, the dialectic between consent and paternalism can be compared with the dialectic between Kantian and utilitarian approaches; in both cases we have, on the one hand, some autonomy condition which is supposed to be necessary for—at least—moral permissibility: the categorical imperative and consent, respectively; and on the other hand we have a utility condition, the utilitarian principle and paternalistic 'best interest' considerations respectively.

So it would be easy to analyse the above cases in terms of the dichotomy between Kantian approaches and utilitarian approaches that we have presented in previous chapters (chapter 3 and chapter 4 respectively); but that still does not deliver us an answer, because could it be that Kant's moral philosophy or deontological theories more in general would really demand that the doctor in the first case lets the patient die and in the second case allows that the foetus either dies or develops serious disabilities? The problem with this conclusion is that it could just as well be taken to constitute a plausible counterexample to Kantian approaches.

On the other hand, one could try to tell a story which would make the case of Joe, say, exceptional: Joe is no longer a minor but he is still very young and has gone through a major traumatic experience at a still young age and, additionally, could be said to be in panic at the moment in which he makes his request for the tube not to be replaced: 'I'd rather die than have that replaced'.

Accordingly, one could add up Joe's youth, his recent traumatic experiences and his current panic together to make a case for the fact that at the moment in which Joe makes his request he is not thinking straight; he could be said to not be in full possession of his autonomous capacities for judgement—and, on these grounds, health professionals may be allowed to take over, so to speak.

It is important to make clear that the above would not mean endorsing utilitarianism or paternalism; after all, alternative approaches too will have to make room for cases when patients are not yet or no longer or just not autonomous: so, for example, children, senile patients affected by neurodegenerative diseases, or patients who are in a temporary state of incapacity, as they may be—say—very drunk or unconscious. In all of these cases, we would not necessarily be taking a paternalistic stand by saying that the patient's wishes must at least be interpreted if not corrected or, indeed, ignored (think of a very drunk patient); it would just be a case of the patient not being in possession of the relevant capacities for autonomous decision making.

This will not work as a general solution, though: first of all because in the cases mentioned above healthcare professionals cannot just decide alone what the best course of action is: they will have to consult family members or other representatives; so that the same paternalistic dilemma could easily be generated by a family member's refusal—from the point of view of healthcare professionals anyway—to decide in the best interest of the patient; just take the case of parents who may be Jehovah's Witnesses and refuse to allow their child to receive a lifesaving blood transfusion.

To this we would have to add the further difficulty of establishing exactly when a patient will count as less than fully autonomous—what do we do with Joe, for example? But this latter problem is not necessarily philosophical in nature, as it could be easily thought that tribunals are the best place for that kind of case-by-case analysis.

One possible solution for this impasse between consent requirements and paternalism could be to say that healthcare professionals take all and only the medical decisions and patients take all and only the personal decisions: after all, the former are the medical experts and the latter are the experts on their own personal situation; so this solution would have clear epistemic advantages.

The problem with this approach is that it is a fiction to believe that we can just sort decisions according to whether they are medical ones or personal ones; just think of the case of Joe: the doctor's decision that the best course of action is replacing the tube could be said to be a medical one, while Joe's insistence that he would rather die than have the tube replaced could be said to be a personal one; even if we could agree on this analysis, it would not bring us forward one bit: exactly because there is a tension between the doctor's medical advice and the patient's personal preferences.

On the other hand, if we accept paternalistic principles, then it is not clear that we can hold on to consent requirements; one hope would be that, instead, by keeping consent requirements and allowing for all the cases where the patient cannot be said to be fully autonomous—because they are too young, and so forth—then we may cover most of the difficult cases; both the cases above, after all, could be dealt with along these lines. And for those intractable cases that are left, we would have to just trust that tribunals will do a good enough job in dealing with the individual intricacies.

This may be, in the end, the most coherent way forward in order not to sacrifice consent requirements within healthcare while at the same time still being able to protect patients and do their best interest; but it would be, obviously, no less than a philosophical retreat, admitting that not all problems can be solved.

To conclude this chapter, we will now briefly present the so-called four principles approach to medical ethics.

The Four Principles

According to the four-principles approach to medical ethics—popularized by Tom Beauchamp and James Childress in their textbook *Principles of Biomedical Ethics*[7]—we can identify four different basic principles that should guide the behaviour of healthcare professionals:

(1) **Autonomy**: *'To respect an autonomous agent is to recognize with due appreciation that person's capacities and perspectives, including his or her right to hold certain views, to make certain choices, and to take certain actions based on personal values and beliefs'*;[8]

(2) **Nonmaleficence**: *primum non nocere (Above all, do no harm)*; *'Blatant examples of failures to act nonmaleficently are found in the use of physicians to classify political dissidents as mentally ill, thereafter treating them with harmful drugs and incarcerating them with insane and violent persons . . . More subtle examples are found in the use of medications for the treatment of aggressive and destructive patients. These common treatment modalities are helpful to many patients, but they can be harmful to others'*;[9]

(3) **Beneficence**: *'The principle of beneficence refers to a moral obligation to act for the benefit of others'*;[10]

(4) **Justice**: *'the minimal (formal) principle that like cases should be treated alike, or, to use the language of equality, equals ought to be treated equally'*.[11]

As the principles are widely known, it is important to comment on them—even though we will see fairly quickly that we have actually already covered all the theoretical issues that are behind those principles: on autonomy and consent we have already said a great deal so we won't go into that.

The same goes, really, also for the harm principle about *nonmaleficience*: but there is one issue that deserves closer attention, namely the fact that the second principle suggests that not doing harm has some sort of priority. Two points here: first, the focus on not *doing* harm suggests that the principle at the same time uses a consequentialist concept—harm—while actually putting forward a nonconsequentialist constraint, namely about what healthcare professionals should not *do*, about their agency. This may be taken to mean that doing harm—as opposed to, say, allowing harm—may be particularly morally problematic—which would be incompatible with consequentialism.

On top of this there is the supposed priority of the nonmaleficience principle: what would that priority imply? This becomes particularly relevant when we move to the third principle about beneficence: does the supposed priority of the second principle imply, for example, that not doing harm is more important, morally speaking, that doing good or helping others? This would be in line with the distinction between negative duties and positive duties but it would—crucially—suggest that we would give priority to the negative duty of not doing harm over the positive duty of help, say.

If we combine the supposed priority of the second principle over the third principle with the nonconsequentialist interpretation of the second principle, we have the so-called *dirty hands* problem: could it be that not getting one's hands dirty—not compromising oneself morally—could be more important than helping people? Surely not; this suggests that we should either interpret the second principle in a consequentialist manner or that we must give up on the priority of the second principle (over the third, say, or in general over the other principles).

Giving up on the priority of the second principle does have its own problems though; as we are then more easily stuck in situations which we cannot resolve in an ethically permissible way, as when we need to do some harm in order to help—a case in which, had the second principle priority over the third—we would at least know what to do; even though, depending on the nature of the help needed, we may be sceptical of whether indeed the second principle should have priority.

These few remarks on the four-principles approach should have sufficed to show—I believe—that actually the issues at stake are the same that we have covered throughout, so that the four principles are not much more than a useful summary—for the healthcare context—of the fundamental ethical principles that we have analysed in this volume. And don't worry, I haven't forgotten about justice: just turn to the next chapter for that.

Summary

Summing up, what we have done in this chapter has been to analyse one of the most important concepts in ethics—consent—which happens to be particularly relevant within the healthcare context; we have discussed both what consent is and what consent can do—with special attention to the limits of consent; this has brought us to the issue of paternalism, namely whether consent is always necessary or whether we can, sometimes, allow healthcare professionals to decide in the best interest of patients. In the last part of the chapter, we then introduced the four principles of medical ethics.

Notes

1. This is from the entry on 'Informed Consent' of the Stanford Encyclopedia of Philosophy: https://plato.stanford.edu/entries/informed-consent/.
2. From Franklin Miller and Alan Wertheimer's *The Ethics of Consent* (Oxford University Press, 2010), 79.
3. Bette-Jane Crigger, *Cases in Bioethics* (New York: Macmillan, 1998).
4. The 'button' is a space holder for a tracheostomy.
5. Crigger, *Cases in Bioethics*, 183.
6. Ibid., 195.
7. Tom Beauchamp and James Childress, *Principles of Biomedical Ethics*, seventh edition (Oxford University Press, 2012).
8. Tom Beauchamp, 'The "Four Principles" Approach to Health Care Ethics', in R. E. Ashcroft, A. Dawson, H. Draper, and J. R. McMillan, eds., *Principles of Health Care Ethics*, second edition (Hoboken, NJ: Wiley, 2007), 4.
9. Ibid., 5.
10. Ibid.
11. Ibid., 6.

CHAPTER SEVEN

Health and Disease

Health(care) Rights and the Value of Health

Health is a good thing—that much we can assume. But what precisely health actually is and exactly how good it is (in comparison to other *goods*, for example) are less obvious questions that this chapter aims to give an answer to. Trying to answer these questions will inevitably confront us with the other side of health, disease.

Those are, in a nutshell, the questions that together amount to the 'value of health' in the title; and they are worth pursuing because to just say that health is valuable will not help us address many practical problems attached to the value of health and, in particular, healthcare: just think of money as a simple example of this. The very question of whether health should be funded publically or privately depends not just on the vague notion of the value of health but on the much more specific issue of how health should be valued in comparison to, well, everything else really—which is what we will be referring to as *other goods*. Also, even if we put aside the huge question of whether healthcare should be funded publically or privately, there will be difficult distributive decisions and choices. Finally, there is the related question of whether healthcare is a human right that should be universally acknowledged—and this last question obviously bears on both the issue of whether healthcare should be publically funded and on distributive principles.

If healthcare is a human right, then that speaks for state-funded coverage, because the entitlement to healthcare would then not depend on how much money someone has or earns. But to establish that healthcare is indeed a right, it won't do to just say that healthcare is valuable; lots of valuable things are not provided for by the state through the public purse but have to be paid for by individuals—just think of ice cream or smartphones.

CASE STUDY I: *Obamacare*

At a time when European healthcare systems are experiencing serious funding problems, due to both cut-downs and rising costs related to an ageing population—while at the same time the Trump administration wants to replace the Affordable Care Act (Obamacare)—the question of the value of health could hardly be more pressing.

A study by the Organisation for Economic Co-operation and Development (OECD) gives a good idea of rising healthcare costs which have outpaced growth in every single member state,[1] showing that the problem is not confined to Europe or the United States (see figure 7.1).

Obviously here healthcare spending is just one simple example of all the different and difficult decisions that are related, both at the level of government and at the level of the private citizen, to health—just think about nutrition, fitness, recreation; most human activities

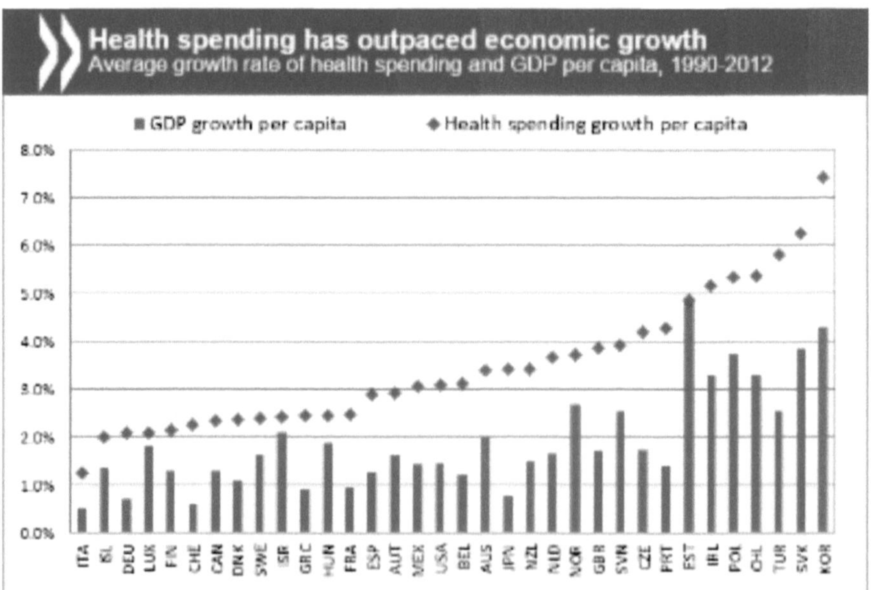

Figure 7.1 Source: OECD (http://www.oecd.org/health/healthcarecostsunsustainableinadvancedeconomieswithoutreform.htm)

have repercussions on health, so that we are making health decisions all the time, whether we are explicitly aware of making them or not.

We will start with the following three hypotheses, the plausibility of which will be tested throughout this chapter:

- Healthcare is a human right (as in, the right to healthcare is universal);
- The value of health is intrinsic;
- Health is the most important good.

All three claims are related to each other but the truth of none of these claims implies the truth of any of the others so that we will have to address all three.

First of all, though, one clarification: we have already distinguished within this book between health and healthcare and this distinction will again be important in this chapter because, for example, it would make no sense to talk outright about a right to health, as our health is not something that we can completely control and disease is often the result of an event over which we had no control; this is the simple reason why, when it comes to rights and ethical questions more in general, it is much more appropriate to address those towards healthcare rather than more broadly towards health—even though obviously in the end it is health that we care about. This is just a version of the familiar 'ought implies can' principle from previous chapters: we can only draw up normative principles for those things that we can control, like healthcare, but not for those things that we cannot control, like health and disease.

Here then is a rough structure that will help us throughout: both health and healthcare are goods but the good (or value) of healthcare depends on the good (or value) of health (while the reverse is clearly not the case). So it is easy to say why healthcare is valuable and a good: because health is valuable and a good. A similar shortcut is not available in the case of health and that is why we need to discuss the question of the value of health in some detail within this chapter.

Finally, it will be beneficial to have a working definition of health as we move forward; for this purpose we will just take the original World Health Organization (WHO) definition from 1948, according to which health is:

> a state of complete physical, mental and social well-being and not merely the absence of disease or infirmity.[2]

This will do for now.[3] As long as the basic difference between healthcare and health is clear and also it is clear that the value of the former depends on the value of the latter, we don't need to say anything else about it here and we can move on to the three hypotheses.

The Right to Health(care)

Let us start with the question of whether healthcare is a human right. If we go back to the principles of the WHO we just referred to, we will see that the WHO certainly thinks that healthcare is a human right:

> The enjoyment of the highest attainable standard of health is one of the fundamental rights of every human being without distinction of race, religion, political belief, economic or social condition.[4]

As we have learned throughout this book, that some person or institution decides that some normative principle applies does not mean that such normative principle actually applies, so that—unfortunately—it is not the WHO that decides whether health is a human right—it is the moral law. The WHO can, at best, institute legal rights, for the justification of which we would then have to appeal to the moral law anyway—so it is the moral law which is the crucial test in any case.

First of all, let us note the small imprecision within the WHO principle due to its appeal to health instead of healthcare. As we have already explained, when it comes to rights, we should more properly talk about healthcare rights instead of health rights simply because of the already familiar 'ought implies can': we can only have normative principles about things that we can do or control—whatever is outside human control is also outside the realm of the moral law; and that applies often in cases of health and disease where there is (still) a lot that we cannot control; the most obvious example of this being the idea—already discussed in chapter 5—that death cannot be prevented or avoided in any meaningful sense but only delayed or postponed.

Still, having put this clarification aside, the question remains of whether people have a human right to healthcare as the WHO suggests. Having distinguished between the right to health and the right to healthcare has the further advantage that we can deal—at least in part—with the idealism of the WHO. Namely, it won't do to just dismiss what the WHO proposes as unrealistic wishful thinking, because once we have translated the WHO proposal in terms of healthcare, that makes it clear that we are only talking about what is humanly possible, namely what the WHO terms 'the highest attainable standard of health'—that is indeed the WHO's way of dealing with the distinction between health and healthcare.

We can now reformulate our question in the following terms: does everybody have the right to the highest attainable standard of health? There are two main issues to deal with here:

- first, the fact that talking in terms of the *highest* standard appears to imply a primacy of health over other goods;
- secondly, that if this is supposed to be a human right then it should apply to people irrespective of their behaviour, which would imply that someone's unhealthy habits, for example, should make no difference to whether and to which extent that person is entitled to healthcare.

Before we look at these two points, an argumentative clarification is called for: the claim that healthcare is a human right does not depend on the claim that every person has a right to the highest attainable standard of health. The right to healthcare could, for example, be less extensive than suggested by the WHO principles—maybe something like a human right to basic healthcare—where that could mean, say, only life-saving care or some such reduced (but maybe more realistic for today's world) standard of care. Here it is not important to be precise about what standard of care we may have a right to, as long as it is clear that there is a difference between arguing for a human right to healthcare and arguing for a human right to the highest attainable standard of health; the latter, as above, may imply a primacy of healthcare over other goods that the former does not imply. Both, though, appear to imply the second point about the right to healthcare being independent from people's behaviour, so we will start from this question.

Some people may believe that quantity and quality of healthcare should at least in part depend on whether the patient has any responsibility for her illness, so that if someone has been reckless and has now become sick as a direct consequence of her recklessness, maybe such a person should not be entitled to as much healthcare as someone who has done everything in her power to avoid becoming sick, for example.

When it comes to luck and responsibility for one's sickness, we can broadly distinguish between the following:

- there are conditions which are as good as unavoidable, as those which are the direct consequence of one's genetic make-up, for example; sometimes people are born with a certain condition, so that there is no way in which we could possibly argue that they themselves are responsible for the condition (even though in some cases it may be possible to make their parents responsible in the relevant way, as in the case in which parents are aware of some serious genetic defect that is very likely to carry on and still decide to reproduce);
- at the other hand of the spectrum, there are conditions which are the direct result of a person's decisions and actions; even though this category is, in theoretical terms, pretty clear, to actually determine which examples will follow under this category is not as easy. So imagine someone that jumps from a window in order to break his own arm so that he will not be conscripted by the military: not only was he aware of the medical effect of his actions but he acted exactly in order to bring about that medical effect, a broken arm.

The case above is pretty straightforward, but you may think that it is not very interesting because it is statistically irrelevant. But there are cases which are, on the other hand, very widespread and of which it is important to determine whether they have the same structure as the broken arm.

CASE STUDY II: Smoking and Drinking

The classics, here, are probably smoking and drinking (but also lack of exercise and poor eating habits may potentially be added to the list). Both habits are demonstrably linked to serious medical conditions; those links have been known for a long time not only within medical circles but within the wider population—and, indeed, both smoking and drinking are becoming less common across Western countries: smoking is down[5]; beer drinking is down[6] (and that applies to alcohol more generally[7]); meat consumption[8] is down too, by the way.

Does smoking work like intentionally breaking one's arm to avoid military conscription? Let me remind the reader why this question is important: we are trying to establish whether there is a right to healthcare; if there is such a right, then people are entitled to healthcare independently from their own intentional behaviour and responsibility. One possible objection to the right to healthcare is reckless behaviour and one of the most widespread cases of such behaviour today could be argued to be smoking.

So we are asking, on the one hand, whether smoking is symmetrical to our thought experiment of intentionally breaking one's arm to avoid military conscription because we are using the latter as a paradigmatic case of a consciously self-inflicted medical condition for which the agent is responsible and we want to know whether smoking and its demonstrable effects should also be dealt with accordingly. On the other hand, we are also asking, ultimately, whether heavy smokers in the twenty-first century should have equal rights to healthcare.

The status of smoking when it comes to individual responsibility is not as simple as the case of intentionally breaking one's arm to avoid military conscription for the following two reasons:

- in the first place, smoking is addictive, so that it would be at least controversial to treat addictive behaviour as equivalent to intentional behaviour[9];
- secondly, smoking is not equally distributed across different social and economic groups: the more disadvantaged someone's background, the more likely they are to smoke; so that it could be argued that smoking is, in some relevant sense, *socially determined* and that therefore at least the most disadvantaged members of our society should not be held responsible for their smoking habits because they are—in brief—a direct result of their poverty or other hardship.[10] Importantly, in this case there is the added complication that if smoking is linked to poverty and we offer less or worse healthcare to smokers, we would be offering less or worse healthcare to the poorest or most deprived, further worsening their situation—and this latter consideration may be considered to be an issue of justice or fairness independently of whether one believes that smokers are responsible for their smoking habit.

The question about smokers' healthcare rights is not just a theoretical one: for example, within Obamacare (the Affordable Care Act), insurers in the United States are allowed to impose higher premiums for smokers of up to 50 percent (even though some states prohibited hikes or capped them at below 50 percent).[11] Interestingly, studies have shown that higher premiums for smokers reduced insurance take-up—making smokers less likely to be insured in the first place—and also did not encourage quitting smoking.[12] So if the whole point of Obamacare was supposed to be to increase the number of Americans with health insurance coverage, then it looks as though allowing insurers to set higher premiums for smokers defeats the very purpose of the Affordable Care Act.[13]

We can debate whether higher premiums are compatible with the rights of smokers—not just their health rights, actually, but nondiscrimination and equality rights more in general; but it seems clear that higher health insurance premiums are not compatible with the letter of the WHO principles, worth restating here in full: 'The enjoyment of the highest attainable standard of health is one of the fundamental rights of every human being without distinction of race, religion, political belief, economic or social condition'.[14]

It is easy to see this by combining two elements of the WHO principles—namely, on the one side, talk of the 'highest attainable standards' and on the other side, talk of 'every human being'—we get a nondiscrimination clause. If every human being is entitled to the highest attainable standard of health, then every human being is entitled—at least—to equal healthcare; indeed, the principle could be easily read in terms of the less-healthy human beings being entitled to more and better healthcare than the healthier human beings, as more and better healthcare will be needed to achieve the highest attainable standard of health for the sick than for the healthy.

The above point is important, as it suggests that WHO principles, in arguing for the highest attainable standard of health for everybody, are actually not just arguing for equal access to healthcare but are rather making—at least implicitly—the case for a progressive access to healthcare, a system in which the sick get more and better healthcare than the healthy—similarly to progressive taxation where, at least in principle, the more you earn the more taxes you pay.

However we interpret WHO principles, anyway, they seem to turn out to be incompatible with higher insurance premiums for smokers, because higher premiums amount to a reduction in access to healthcare for smokers. So when it comes to smoking we seem to face the following alternative: on the one hand, equal health rights would suggest that smokers should be given at least the same access to healthcare that is granted to nonsmokers, so that higher premiums would be illegitimate.

On the other hand, the case of smokers could be used to argue against the human right to the highest attainable standard of health. And indeed the case of higher premiums for smokers may just show that the whole system of private health insurance is not compatible with healthcare as a human right.

A clarification is called for: higher premiums for smokers are not only incompatible with WHO principles—which some readers may consider radically progressive or too optimistic; higher premiums for smokers appear to be incompatible also with a more moderate version of healthcare rights which does not appeal to the 'highest attainable standard of health'. We have actually already seen this point: whether we talk of the highest attainable standard of health or alternatively of some more basic level of healthcare, the point of using the human rights language is that, then, healthcare rights would be universal whatever their content—and it is their universality, as we have seen above, that would prohibit distinguishing between smokers and nonsmokers the way in which higher insurance premiums do.

This is not the place to resolve these complicated issues about the causes and circumstances of smoking. It is enough that we have illustrated what the first argument against a universal right to healthcare amounts to: bad habits such as smoking or heavy drinking would have to be considered intentional actions for which agents are responsible—and we have seen at least two kinds of considerations against this view. But that alone would not be enough: even if chain smoking and heavy drinking were to be equivalent to intentionally breaking one's arm in order to avoid conscription so that agents would be responsible for the resulting medical conditions, we would still be missing an additional normative premise according to which when patients are responsible for their medical conditions, then they are not entitled to healthcare or anyway they are not entitled to the same healthcare they would have been entitled to had they not been responsible for their medical condition (these two are obviously very different in outcome but for present argumentative purposes we can deal with them together).

What would be the ethical reason for thinking that if a patient is responsible for their medical condition, then they are not entitled to (equal) healthcare? The following may be a plausible candidate: healthcare is an important good; if someone forfeits such good intentionally by disregarding their value, why should everyone else have to contribute to try to correct such recklessness?

CASE STUDY III: A Hiking Trip

You may compare this to the following little story: you and your friends have set out early on a long hiking trip; everybody has the same amount (and quality) of food at the beginning of the trip; your friend Emma can't be bothered with the extra weight of her food portion so she left it behind at the beginning of the hike; when you pause to eat Emma is clearly hungry; should everyone else now chip in (thereby reducing their own food portion) so that Emma gets something to eat, even though she originally had just as much and intentionally (and freely) left it behind? Remember, I am not comparing this little story to smoking or any other habit with negative consequences for health, as we have already discussed how difficult such comparisons would be. Here we are only interested in the principle behind the idea that, if someone is responsible for their needy situation, then they should not be entitled to as much as everyone else—so that we could compare Emma not just with everyone else who has carried the extra weight but also with Laura, whose food has been stolen along the way, we may suppose.

Would it be fair to distinguish between Emma and Laura when it comes to distributing whatever food resources are available? Or even more radically: would it not be unfair to give Emma the same amount of food we give to Laura, given that the former's need is self-inflicted while the latter's need is not her responsibility?

In this context political philosophers often speak of so-called *luck egalitarianism*, according to which distributive principles should only take into account differences for which agents are responsible and disregard differences which are the result of pure luck.[15]

Whatever we think about the plausibility of the hiking trip scenario and the way in which it should be compared with real life (after all, it is plausible to imagine that, within any group of friends, some people will find hiking more challenging than others, for example), our little thought experiment makes clear that we should think of healthcare along the lines of one of the vital resources (indeed, *goods*) the distribution of which needs to be regulated by ethical, legal, and political principles, like money (and indeed *health* and *wealth* even sound similar, and money could be considered to be the vehicle of wealth the way in which here we have been thinking of healthcare as the vehicle of health).

The Value of Health

This brings us to the other possible objection to the WHO principle according to which everyone has a right to the highest attainable standard of health, namely the question of whether health has some sort of priority over other distributable resources; that is, by the way, where the issue of the right to healthcare crosses with the other two issues we have identified at the beginning of this chapter: whether health is the highest good and whether its value is intrinsic.

These questions are themselves both difficult and important but they also throw up, I think, an even more fundamental question about the role of ethics and values within a liberal society. In very simple terms: when it comes to the value of health—both in itself and in comparison to other goods—who should decide, at least in a liberal context? Is the value of health even an ethical issue?

To put it differently: in a liberal and open society, shouldn't every individual be able to decide how important health is to them? So that the question about the value of health would not belong inside an ethics book. If you reflect upon what we have discussed so far within this chapter, you will see that this question is not as straightforward as it may appear: because on the one hand, we might be tempted to be as liberal as possible about the value of health so that everyone should be able to decide for themselves how important health is to them; but on the other hand, we may also be tempted to be as progressive as possible and defend everyone's human right to healthcare. Both those positions are *liberal* ones in the modern (American) sense of liberal; but are these two positions compatible? Can we, simultaneously, defend the human right to the highest attainable level of health (or some more moderate human right to healthcare) while also leave it to every individual to decide how important health (and therefore healthcare) is to them?

This tension goes to the heart of the question about the value of health and healthcare: if health is so important as to be a universal human right, then shouldn't its value be—at least to some extent—independent of how different individuals rate it? Here the reader should not be surprised to see, again, some of the same questions that came up in previous chapters surface again for the case of the value of health:

- Is the value of health objective or subjective?
- Is health intrinsically valuable?
- How does the value of health compare to the values of other goods?

Besides the above questions we have the broader political issue of how liberal societies should deal with values, whether it is the value of health or some other value. Some of the relevant problems, here, have already been dealt with in the chapter about life and death: life is, after all, also a case in which we want to say, on the one hand, that the right to life is a universal human right but also be liberal about the value that different individuals will attach to it, see the discussion of suicide and euthanasia in chapter 5.

Let us be brutally clear here: can we normatively legislate that it is either morally wrong or irrational to disvalue or disregard health and healthcare? Here we should distinguish between disregarding the value of health and healthcare for others—which can constitute both harm and an autonomy violation—and disregard the value of one's own health. This distinction easily applies to one's children as well, so that parents can be and should be made responsible for bad health choices on behalf of their children: think of recent debates on vaccination, for example; but also, even more straightforwardly, think of cases in which parents disregard a doctor's advice or if they miss doctors' appointments for their children.

Still, even in the relatively easy case of the parent–child relationship, the question about the value of health is crucial: just compare this to education. Even though most countries have at least a number of years in which school is obligatory for children, there are exceptions for home-schooling one's children and there is also a great degree of parental autonomy in terms of educational choices. How much of that kind of parental autonomy should also be appropriate to health choices will depend on the value of health. Can we oblige parents, for example, not to feed their children ready-meals? Can we prohibit parents from giving their children fizzy drinks? And what about candy?

CASE STUDY IV: My Daughter's Muesli

Those issues are not just complicated in practice: these problems are principled ones. So for example, aren't parents best placed to make a health/happiness trade-off on behalf of their children? That is, if you like, what parents do all the time in deciding how often how much candy a child can have. Take my daughter, who woke up this morning wanting candy for breakfast instead of the muesli which I had already prepared and that she usually eats for breakfast. Aren't my wife and I best placed to decide whether or not to make an exception? My daughter may, after all, have had a bad dream or a tough time at school the day before, and so on. More crucially for the purposes of this chapter, whether or not to make an exception (assuming that candy for breakfast on a regular basis is really a no go, which it is!) will again depend on the value of health.

This anecdote serves multiple purposes (by the way, we did not make an exception and my daughter did not get candy for breakfast; unfortunately she didn't eat her muesli either and went to school on an empty stomach): first, it shows how difficult it would be, both in theory and in practice, to defend and implement the idea that the value of health has priority over everything else, so that in every case we should decide against a health trade-off; whether it is ourselves, our children, or the healthcare system as a whole, it is not even clear what a world in which we always decided against health trade-offs would look like—even though I may be permitted to say that some health-obsessed areas of some Scandinavian capital I won't name might be starting to give us a clue about what that particular dystopia would look like!

Clearly, though, the idea that disregarding the value of health is either morally or rationally problematic does not have to be implemented to the extreme degree of never making health trade-offs. Still, the extreme cases of never allowing your children candy or, say, going for a run every single day cannot be easily dismissed if we don't get some clarity on the value of health—and the very same considerations will apply to more radical cases such as smoking and what treatment smokers deserve.

Here someone may get worried that we are confusing the right to health with a duty to be healthy: after all, we could easily formulate matters in terms of the state or healthcare system giving everybody equal access to healthcare without at the same time thereby coercing anyone into taking advantage of their healthcare services. This piece of common sense is plausible, but it is unfortunately not very helpful: first of all, it does not say on which grounds the state should grant everybody equal access to healthcare nor does it say what that equal access should amount to. After all, as we saw at the beginning of this chapter, healthcare ain't cheap; on the contrary: a commitment to equal access to a good standard of healthcare for every citizen is a big investment.

Data shows that OECD countries on average spend around 9 percent of GDP on healthcare, with the United States spending as much as 17 percent.[16] According to these measures from the World Bank, Denmark spends just below 11 percent.[17]

What the above piece of common sense also does not say is what we should do with those who disvalue health: smokers and heavy drinkers, for example—but even a coherent way of formulating this list is difficult; what about unhealthy eaters or those who do no exercise, or even just habitual risk takers (say, bungee jumping once a week)? If health is so important that modern states can be reasonably expected to spend a substantial part of their budget on it, then do we have reason to mandate health, thereby coercing healthy habits (independently of whether that works, as we have seen that it does not work with smokers in the United States)? It is time to at least try to give some answers: here I am going to focus on two different answers, a more formal one if you like and a more substantial (and inevitably tentative) one, starting from the latter.

Health as a Means to Life's Ends

We should not overestimate health. After all, whatever its value (and tellingly, at least its perceived value tends to vary depending on how sick or healthy a person is at a certain time), health is hardly ever one of life's achievements or goals. If you ask people what they want to achieve in life or what their goals are, it would be very strange to hear them answer that their life goal is to be healthy. This is obviously culturally dependent and it also changes over time (both through history but also over a lifetime, presumably), and still it may be more plausible to think of health as a necessary condition or a facilitator for whatever we want to achieve in life. In philosophical terms, then, what I am arguing for could be easily formulated in terms of health being not an end but a means to life's ends.

This proposal is arguably at odds with the idea that health is intrinsically valuable: after all, a standard understanding of 'intrinsic' value is value that does not depend on anything else; and if we understand health as a means to life's ends, then the value of health would itself depend on the value of the ends that health allows us to achieve. And this is, indeed, what I think is the most plausible understanding of the value of health: that its value depends on what health allows us to achieve does not mean, by the way, that health is not very valuable; as it is easy to see that, without health, we could hardly achieve anything, then we can also see that even though it is just a means to life's ends, health is nonetheless very valuable because life's ends are valuable and they could not be achieved if we were not healthy.

This proposal is already very tentative so I don't want to go too far but I will say that, when you think about it, if you find the above argument plausible for the case of health, you may also find it similarly plausible for the case of life itself. This comparison allows me to make a clarification: talk of life's ends which are enabled by health might give the impression that I am restricting this to ends and goals we can achieve in terms of what we can *do*; but that would be a mistake, as very often what is valuable and what health enables are nonagential events upon which we have no control, as for example, seeing our children grow up. If I had to say today what was the main reason why I want to be and hope to be healthy, I would have no doubt that it would be to see my children grow up; and even though that is something upon which we can have a great degree of influence, it is certainly not our *action* in any traditional sense nor should it ever be considered to be *our* achievement as parents. In this respect life's goals of which health is a crucial enabler should be understood in this broader nonagential way.

On the negative side of things, the very same argument applies to suffering and death: those are not actions of ours in any traditional sense, but just as health can be considered to be an enabler for life's goals it can be equally considered to be an avoider of suffering and death and thereby again a means rather than an end in itself.

Understanding health as a means to life's ends gives an answer to the other two of the three questions that we posed at the beginning of this chapter, as it rules out—for the reasons we have just seen—the idea that health is intrinsically valuable; and it also speaks against the idea that health is the most important of life's goods; indeed, on this view it would be more plausible to think of the ends that are enabled by health as the most important goods (however we are in the end going to interpret 'important').

At this stage we should also introduce what at the beginning of this section I referred to as a more formal answer to the question of the value of health: after all, to think of health as a means still does not tell us how valuable health is and who should adjudicate the value of health—which are clearly the most important and interesting questions at least from a practical point of view. By now, though, it should be clear that we don't need an answer to these questions here because these questions may be ultimately philosophical but they are not purely ethical questions. The value of health depends on the ends it enables: and the value of these ends that health enables (be that love, happiness, seeing one's children grow up or, more mundanely, fame and riches) is something that a liberal society leaves up to its citizens, so that everyone should be entitled to their own conception of the good and correspondingly to the particular place that health and healthcare will occupy within their conception of the good.[18]

I would understand if the reader were a bit disappointed by this outcome: we are still to resolve the tension between health(care) rights on the one hand and the liberal value of health on the other. If we are entitled to some degree of healthcare as a matter of human rights, then that entitlement will have to be taken into account in any distributive decision, no matter what members of a liberal society agree in terms of how important health will be to them collectively.

This is an important point which allows us to reconnect the two directions that this chapter has taken: on the one hand, we have discussed the issue of health rights and especially whether there is a human right to healthcare. On the other hand, we have discussed what the value of health should be. What we have learned throughout this book should now allow us to better understand this tension: it is only about the latter issue that we can be confidently liberal; because if there are health rights, the existence of those rights does not necessarily depend on whether society agrees to respect them; health rights, just like moral rights, may have an independent normative force (as in, independent from whether or not people or societies endorse them).

We cannot resolve all of these difficult issues here: it will have to be enough to have made some progress in understanding what the problems and possible solutions are. In the end, we can hold on to at least the following: health(care) rights, if they exist, are positive rights against the state or other people to receive healthcare. Even if there is such a thing as health rights, that does not mean that anybody should be coerced into healthy behaviour or prohibited from unhealthy behaviour, because a liberal society should respect everybody's own conception of how valuable health is to them.

Still, we have identified a tension between health rights on the one hand and a liberal conception of the value of health, so that it is difficult to answer distributive questions about how much healthcare any given individual should be entitled to: at the extremes of this distributive tension we have identified, on the one hand, the progressive principle from the WHO according to which everybody is entitled to the highest attainable standard of health and at the other extreme the idea that there are no health entitlements and that healthcare should be left to market forces just like any other industry: just the way in which it is up to you and you alone to decide how much a new car is worth to you, it should be up to you and you alone to decide how much some treatment is worth to you.

Public vs. Private Healthcare

As in many other instances throughout this book, I am afraid that again in this chapter I have not managed to provide concrete answers to the difficult practical and political questions which depend upon the principles we have analysed. A particularly controversial example, within the context of this chapter, is clearly the issue of whether healthcare should be publicly funded: we have shown the link between this political question and the philosophical issue of whether healthcare is a human right but we have not actually answered the former—political—question. So in this section I will briefly address that.

First of all, we should clarify what the question regarding public healthcare amounts to: it is, if you like, a question about who should pay for healthcare rather than a question about whether healthcare should be free of charge, as in systems in which healthcare is publicly funded it is paid for through taxation or mandatory health insurance (which still amounts to the same, namely deductions from your income); so it may seem that healthcare has to be paid for no matter what and that the question is only who should shoulder the burden, so to speak.

But we will see that, actually, there are at least two different questions here: on the one hand there is the question of who should pay—which is really the question of whether one should be entitled to healthcare coverage even if one cannot afford it and whether healthcare coverage should be equal for everybody independently of income. But there is also another—possibly less obvious—question: namely, the issue of whether one should be obliged to contribute to their country's healthcare expenditure, through taxation or mandatory health insurance.

From an ethical point of view, it is interesting to note how these two questions are about rights and duties: should you be entitled to (equal) healthcare coverage even if you cannot afford it? That is a question about a positive right that every citizen would have against the rest of the collective. Should you be obliged to contribute to your collective's healthcare expenses? That is a question about a positive duty that every member of the collective would have. And it is clearly the positive duty which would guarantee and cover for the positive right, so those two questions are related: as we have already learned, the relevant positive right would be empty without its corresponding positive duty.

This will have hopefully further clarified why it was so important to discuss in some detail the value of healthcare as we did in this chapter—because if the collective is not obliged to contribute, then the individual right to healthcare cannot be respected. But on what grounds should the collective be obliged to contribute if healthcare were not valuable in a way such as to warrant a positive duty to value it?

Still, we have not answered the practical question: should healthcare be publically funded and available to everyone irrespective of their income? At this political level, it is important to distinguish between the question of whether healthcare should be accessible to everyone irrespective of income (which is the practical placeholder for what we have said about individual responsibility throughout this chapter) and the question of whether everybody should be entitled to the same amount and quality of healthcare; this latter question also has bearing on the related issue of whether private coverage should even be permitted within healthcare, as many European countries have systems in which there is a basket of healthcare services guaranteed to everyone while at the same time allowing citizens to pay extra—privately—for further (or better) healthcare services.

CASE STUDY V: *Private Schools*

This is like private school: in most developed countries, a place in a public school (as in, state school) is guaranteed to everyone but parents are also free—if they want to—to pay for private school for their children.

In both the education and healthcare debate, we may ask whether these kinds of freedoms are legitimate. And this latter question is related to the question of equal access to healthcare and education, as allowing for private healthcare and education—even in a system in which there is a guaranteed minimum of education and healthcare for everyone irrespective of income—does in the end mean, at least in practice, that there will not be equal education or healthcare; and indeed, it would be difficult even to insist that there would be, in these circumstances, equal access to education and healthcare, as the majority would not have access to private healthcare and education, thereby making access to healthcare and education not equal.

Still, if we want to be liberal about the value of health, the discussion within this chapter should have also shown the problems with not allowing for private health coverage on top of the publicly funded basket. If every citizen should be left the freedom to decide how important healthcare is to them, then supposedly that should also mean that we should allow citizen to invest the rest of their income on further healthcare services if they so wish—but this does have the unwelcome consequence, for many anyway, that we thereby sacrifice equal access to healthcare.

Unsurprisingly, you will have noticed that this debate has the same structure of other philosophical and political debates about freedom and distribution of resources, so that it is extremely difficult to argue that a perfectly equal society—whether we talk of equal outcomes or only equal opportunities—is a perfectly liberal society as well; here we would quickly get into intricate issues in political philosophy and political theory which are out of place here; for the interested reader I recommend that they start from the modern classic on these issues, John Rawls's *A Theory of Justice*. It is worth noting, for example, that Rawls in *A Theory of Justice* lists health as a primary good, a natural primary good—as opposed to social primary goods; primary goods are, according to Rawls, 'things which it is supposed a rational man wants whatever else he wants'.[19]

A final thought on how these debates bear on healthcare: perfectly equal access to healthcare coverage without allowing for any private involvement may have been easier to defend had the value of healthcare been intrinsic, because there would have been good reason against any kind of difference and discrimination; so that here we see how another of the main contentions of this chapter—the question of whether or not the value of healthcare should be considered to be intrinsic—has direct bearing on the political consequences for healthcare.

That in the end we may have to allow some room for private enterprise within healthcare does not mean—mind you—that we should not be careful in controlling and monitoring private involvement in healthcare. A particularly worrying development, in this respect, is currently the way in which technological progress and innovation in healthcare is implicitly making more room for private enterprise by making healthcare services both more expensive and more complicated.

Even though, clearly, we should not be blind to the amazing new clinical possibilities that innovation in healthcare is allowing for, we should be careful that the increased *technologizing* of healthcare does not also deliver, with it, the increased privatizing of healthcare: that ought to be a political decision and a political decision alone, not a technological or bureaucratic one.

Disability

We have been assuming throughout this chapter that health is a good thing (and consequently that its opposite, disease, is a negative) and have rather focused on how good it is and whether it is a matter of rights. In this last section I am going to address a possible objection (or at least exception) to the assumption that health is a good thing: disability.

To put the issue in simple terms: is disability a bad thing or are we just living in a massively ableist world?[20] First of all, a clarification: where does disability fit within the health/disease dichotomy? It should not be assumed that a disabled person is unhealthy, for example.[21] On the other hand, would you rather have been born with a certain disability or without it? Would you rather have been born blind or sighted, say?

CASE STUDY VI: Preterm Babies

Difficult choices depend on the value of disability: would you abort a foetus which had been found to have a serious genetic condition? And what about something not as serious, like Down Syndrome? Another difficult case is represented by preterm babies: 'Human viability, defined as gestational age at which the chance of survival is 50%, is currently approximately 23–24 weeks in developed countries . . . Despite technological advances and efforts of child health experts during the last generation, the extremely premature infant (less than 28 weeks gestation) and extremely low birth weight infant (ELBW) (< 1000 grams) remain at high risk for death and disability with 30–50% mortality and, in survivors, at least 20–50% risk of morbidity'.[22] So these questions about the value of disability are not just theoretical questions but have practical consequences both for healthcare professionals and patients (including parents and perspective parents).

You may think that the question I am addressing here is weird: obviously, disability is a negative, you may say; who in their right mind would ever *want* to be disabled or not prefer not having been disabled? But—if you reflect upon it—you may see that this reaction could also just be the result of living in an ableist world. After all, what is the problem with disability? One obvious problem, in our societies, is that disabled people are at a massive disadvantage in terms of what they can do, experience, achieve. Why are disabled people at such great disadvantage? It could be that this is because, for any given disability, a disabled person is living in a world where the majority of people are not disabled in that particular respect so that the majority has structured society according to the needs of the nondisabled instead of according to the needs of the disabled. That is ableism: discrimination against disabled people.

Is it even possible to imagine, though, a world in which being blind would be better or at least not worse than being sighted? And if we can't, is that a failure of the imagination or an argument in favour of the idea that disability is not socially constructed? This debate is, if nothing else, an important reminder of how massively biased towards nondisabled people our world is; and, if I might add, of the fact that such bias is, for the most part, an economic one. After all, lots of people including myself wear spectacles. Why don't we consider people with spectacles as disabled? Is it just because spectacles have become so cheap and readily available? That would just go to show that the disadvantages connected to disability depend on having failed to structure society (homes, cities, transport, etc.) around the needs of the disabled instead of around the needs of the nondisabled.

The spectacle example is also a good reminder of how difficult it is to establish what should count as a disability; so that even if not all disability is socially constructed, it is certainly the case that some conditions may cease to count as disabilities through progress and technological innovation.

This is not the place to properly engage with this debate so I will just briefly summarize its dialectic structure: at the one theoretical extreme is the view that disability is a natural disadvantage while at the other theoretical extreme is the view that disability is socially constructed and that all disadvantages linked to it are merely the result of the nondisabled majority having structured society according to its own interests while disregarding the needs of those with disabilities.

In between, there are serious equality considerations about the rights of people with disabilities and the fight against ableism; luckily enough, those considerations of equality for people with disabilities do not necessarily depend on endorsing the idea that all disadvantages are social ones; it could be, for example, that a blind person is at a natural disadvantage in comparison with a sighted person because of all the beautiful things that the former person cannot see and that, all the same, we are ethically required to structure society so as to guarantee equal opportunities for the disabled person or at least so as to reduce disadvantages as much as possible—this does not sound at all like a radical idea, however expensive it may be.

Why—to conclude—this brief digression on the issue of disability? It serves as an illustration of two of the important issues in this chapter: the implications of assuming that health is valuable and the difficulty in determining exactly what is the value of health. In particular, the latter is an important reminder of how difficult distributive decisions are within healthcare and beyond: how much are we willing to spend in order to give disabled people equal opportunity is just another version of the question how expensive is too expensive for some new cancer medication. As often with philosophy, theoretical debates massively underestimate the intricacies on the ground but hopefully we have made a helpful start in answering some of these difficult questions.

Summary

In this chapter, we have analysed the value of health—addressing for example the question of whether there is a human right to healthcare and what such a right would amount to. We have then illustrated the implications of this theoretical questions for many current political debates—for example, the rights and duties of smokers within a liberal society and the question of whether healthcare should be publicly funded. The chapter concludes with a brief discussion of the topic which emphasizes the intricacies around health and disease and the value of health: disability.

Notes

1. http://www.oecd.org/health/healthcarecostsunsustainableinadvancedeconomies withoutreform.htm.

2. http://www.who.int/about/mission/en/.

3. For a more detailed discussion of the concepts of health and disease, see the relevant *Stanford Encyclopedia of Philosophy* article: https://plato.stanford.edu/entries/health -disease/.

4. http://www.who.int/about/mission/en/.

5. http://csi.nuff.ox.ac.uk/?p=390.

6. http://www.ias.org.uk/Alcohol-knowledge-centre/Consumption/Factsheets/Total-consumption-in-the-UK.aspx#_edn1.

7. http://www.newstatesman.com/politics/health/2015/10/strange-death-boozy-britain-why-are-young-people-drinking-less.

8. https://www.theguardian.com/news/datablog/2013/jun/05/meat-consumption-uk-global-trends.

9. On action and addiction, see for example my own article 'Addiction, Compulsion and Agency', *Neuroethics* 7, no. 1 (2014): 105–07, doi:10.1007/s12152–013–9184-x and also the article to which mine reacts: H. Pickard, 'The purpose in chronic addiction', *AJOB Neuroscience* 3, no. 2 (2012): 40–49, doi: 10.1080/21507740.2012.663058.

10. On this point see, for example, K. Grill and K. Voigt, 'The Case for Banning Cigarettes', *Journal of Medical Ethics* 42 (2016): 293–301, available at: http://jme.bmj.com/content/42/5/293.

11. http://content.healthaffairs.org/content/35/7/1176.abstract.

12. See again http://content.healthaffairs.org/content/35/7/1176.abstract, and also see the following *HuffPost* article for a good nonacademic summary of the findings: http://www.huffingtonpost.com/entry/obamacare-smokers-study_us_577d3de2e4b0a629c1ab828a.

13. The reader may be curious to find out what counts as a smoker for the purpose of allowed higher premiums within Obamacare. Here's the answer: 'the use of a tobacco product or products four or more times per week within no longer than the past 6 months'. https://www.cms.gov/CCIIO/Resources/Files/Downloads/market-rules-technical-summary-2–27–2013.pdf.

14. http://www.who.int/about/mission/en/.

15. For a good overall discussion of luck egalitarianism, see Kasper Lippert-Rasmussen's book, *Luck Egalitarianism* (London: Bloomsbury, 2016). For a discussion of luck egalitarianism which is applied to issues within healthcare, see Shlomi Segall's book, *Health, Luck, and Justice* (Princeton, NJ: Princeton University Press, 2009).

16. http://visual.ons.gov.uk/how-does-uk-healthcare-spending-compare-internationally/. It is important to clarify that those numbers include both public and private expenditure: that explains why the United States spends so much, one may argue; for a more detailed split between public and private expenditure, please see the link above.

17. http://data.worldbank.org/indicator/SH.XPD.TOTL.ZS?locations=DK&year_high_desc=true.

18. Conception of the good is a somewhat technical term that I am borrowing from Rawls, see here for more details: https://plato.stanford.edu/entries/original-position/.

19. John Rawls, *A Theory of Justice* (Cambridge, MA: Harvard University Press, 1971), 179.

20. For an introduction to this issue, see https://plato.stanford.edu/entries/disability/ and for an interesting instance of this debate see www.journals.uchicago.edu/doi/abs/10.1086/677021 and http://www.journals.uchicago.edu/doi/full/10.1086/684709.

21. On this issue, see https://link.springer.com/article/10.1007/s10677–016–9735–4.

22. https://www.ncbi.nlm.nih.gov/pmc/articles/PMC4438860/.

CHAPTER EIGHT

Praise and Blame

Responsibility and Liability in Healthcare

In this final chapter, we shall discuss an ethical issue which has been implicit within most of what we have said so far: responsibility. There are many different ways in which the concept of responsibility is crucial to healthcare: we have just seen in the previous chapter one such way, namely the question of whether the fact that a patient can be deemed to have been responsible for her medical condition should be taken into consideration when making decisions about the distribution of healthcare resources; and in that context, with the example of smokers, we have also already had a taste of how difficult it is to answer the question of whether someone is responsible for some action of his, given both the addictive character of smoking and the fact that smoking seems to depend on your social and economic situation.

We already know, then, that responsibility is both relevant to healthcare and a complex issue. There are also other obvious ways in which responsibility is relevant to healthcare: one is, for example, the question of under what conditions doctors and other healthcare professionals should be held responsible for some error, mistake and, in the extreme case, for having done something wrong—and here along with responsibility the relevant concepts will be blame, accountability, and liability.

A further question related to the issue of responsibility within healthcare is whether healthcare professionals should be thought of as having a particular kind of responsibility, which might, for example, depend on the particular knowledge, skills, and also power that they acquire. Does—in a slogan—greater power or knowledge also mean increased responsibility?

What we will try to do in this chapter is to make some progress in understanding the concept of responsibility: what does it mean to be responsible or, which is the same, under what conditions is someone responsible for some action or event? We will address this question both in general and in its application to healthcare; and in doing so we will hopefully come closer to giving some answers to the questions above.

To begin with though, let us make clear that there is a classic debate around moral responsibility that we will ignore within this chapter, namely the issue of free will and whether we can only be morally responsible if the world is not causally determined. We have talked about determinism in chapter 1 and we will not expand on that debate here—so that our discussion of responsibility will bypass, in as far as it is possible, the question of how we should understand free will and whether it is compatible with moral responsibility. Terminologically speaking, we will use 'responsibility' instead of 'moral responsibility' exactly so as to distinguish what we discuss in this chapter from the issue of free will.

Having set free will aside, the chapter will be structured around the following three topics:

1) Conditions for responsibility
2) Mistakes and responsibility
3) Special responsibility

The next section will cover the first two issues while the section after next will discuss whether healthcare professionals have any sort of special responsibility.

Conditions for Responsibility and Mistakes

The first question is basically the following:

Under what conditions is an agent responsible for what she does?

Here we should first clarify that even though we are using the word 'responsibility' in an unqualified way to distinguish our use from the 'moral responsibility' of the free-will debate, there is still an important distinction to be drawn between being morally responsible and being legally responsible; so that it is indeed possible both that someone is morally responsible without being legally responsible and also that someone is legally responsible without being morally responsible—*strict liability* may be a case of the latter for example.

Before analysing the conditions for responsibility, it may be beneficial to ask the obvious question of why responsibility is important. The answer is that beings like ours distinguish between events that have been brought about by other agents and events that have happened naturally or by accident without the agential involvement of other people. So, for example, it makes a difference to us whether an injury was the result of bad luck or whether it was the result of, say, an unfair tackle on the football pitch.

It makes, first of all, a difference in the way in which we relate to other people on a personal level; but it obviously also makes a difference in the way in which our society is structured (just think of the consequences for an insurance company of whether the injury was a freak accident or whether it was caused by another player, for example); finally, it makes a difference in terms of the law and questions of punishment within the legal system. So whether or not we can attribute some event to another agent matters to us and therefore it matters to us if and when people are responsible.

Indeed, it has been suggested (prominently by P. F. Strawson in *Freedom and Resentment*) that responsibility is not just important but a part of who we are, namely beings who can't help but hold each other responsible. In what follows, I will take the value of being able to hold each other responsible in a consistent and coherent way as a given and analyse possible principles according to which we may be able to do that.

To start with, we should acknowledge the difference between what merely *happens* and what we *do*—normally within philosophy people speak of events as opposed to actions (Donald Davidson, for example, has argued that actions are a type of event, so that all actions are events but not all events are actions[1]). But here we cannot take the shortcut of just arguing that all and only actions are the events that we are responsible for and that all events which are not actions we are not responsible for. We will see that matters are more complicated than this, even though it is natural to think that, normally, we are responsible for our actions and also that there are many events which are not actions and that we are—therefore—not responsible for.

Both these basic principles have exceptions but we can start from there. If you miss an appointment because a thunderstorm has caused a traffic jam, we are normally going to take it that you are not responsible for missing the appointment—the storm just happened and it was not something that can be attributed to you. Sure, matters start to sound a bit different if it was the case that, say, there had been plenty of advance warning and you had been advised against driving because of the incoming storm but you still decided to drive and got stuck in traffic instead of safely arriving at your appointment in time by, say, taking the metro.

Still, storms are normally things that we do not attribute to agents, who are the victims (not the perpetrators) of storms—this is where often the law speaks of *force majeure*. The idea would be that—under certain conditions—the storm is a good enough excuse for your missing the appointment so that you are not responsible for missing the appointment.

CASE STUDY I: *Federer*

Now contrast this case with a case in which you missed the appointment because there was a tennis match on telly that you did not want to miss (Roger Federer, let us stipulate!) We may speak as though Federer prevented you from making the appointment the way in which the storm also prevented you from making the appointment but, clearly, the two cases are completely different, so that in this new case you decided not to go to the appointment because you preferred watching Federer. Whether or not that was a wise choice will depend on other issues (had the appointment been an important health check, for example, then watching Federer may have been unwise; but maybe it was just a school reunion to which watching Federer can understandably be preferred). That's irrelevant, though, to the issue of responsibility: whatever your reasons, you are responsible for missing the appointment in the case in which you decide to stay at home and watch Federer—that's an intentional action of yours which is the result of a voluntary and autonomous decision, so it's a no brainer.

Things become more difficult in the following case: suppose the appointment is a work-related meeting and the reason why you miss it is to pick up your kid from school after they phoned you to say she was not feeling well. In this case it sounds like you are still responsible for missing the appointment—missing it is no accident but a voluntary decision of yours—but this time missing the appointment seems to be a reasonable choice for which you cannot be blamed; you were not just excused from the appointment given your daughter's sickness, you were actually justified in choosing to pick up your sick daughter over going to the appointment.

Justification, Excuse and Mitigating Considerations

We have already learned something important here: blame and responsibility can easily come apart as in the above case, in which we can still hold you responsible for not showing up at the meeting even though you are blameless because it was not only understandable but also justified that you preferred picking up your sick daughter from school (on this and related issues, I recommend H. L. A. Hart's *Punishment and Responsibility*[2]). In the philosophy of law, it is common to distinguish—following Hart—between:

a) Justification
b) Excuse
c) Mitigation

In the 'Prolegomenon to the Principles of Punishment', Hart writes that:

> In the case of 'justification' what is done is regarded as something which the law does not condemn, or even welcomes. But where killing (e.g. accidental) is excused, criminal responsibility is excluded on a different footing. What has been done is something which is deplored, but the psychological state of the agent when he did it exemplified one or more of a variety of conditions which are held to rule out the public condemnation and punishment of individuals . . . The most prominent of these excusing conditions are those forms of lack of knowledge which make action unintentional: lack of muscular control which makes it involuntary, subjection to gross forms of coercion by threats, and types of mental abnormality, which are believed to render the agent incapable of choice or of carrying out what he has chosen to do.[3]

Hart goes on to clarify that, despite their differences, justification and excuse have in common that they rule out conviction and punishment; that is what distinguishes them both from mitigation, which presupposes conviction and liability and where the question is the nature of the punishment. This is also where Hart's other distinction between *convicting* and *sentencing* is crucial: while justification and excuse belong to the phase of convicting someone, mitigation belongs to the later phase of sentencing someone once she has already been convicted (within a criminal trial, that is).

CASE STUDY II: *The Neglected Patient*

Let us bring these distinctions back to healthcare by reflecting upon the following case: a nurse is forced to neglect a patient who is requesting her presence because another patient—which she judges as more urgently requiring care—has just been brought in. The nurse's behaviour is justified: we can still attribute the neglect to her in the sense that she has made a call to prioritize a patient over the other but there is no blame attached to that.

Alternatively, we may imagine that what explains the neglect is that the nurse has been doing double shifts, has not been off the last eighteen hours, and she is too tired to notice the red light from the patient's room. Again, it seems that the nurse is blameless because an eighteen-hour shift is a good enough excuse and, presumably, not her fault. But the nurse's behaviour is still, at least in principle, one that we want to condemn—it is just that the circumstances are such that we ought not to condemn the nurse for it.

Both of the above cases should be distinguished from a case in which the nurse is so distracted and nervous—because she is expecting news from her daughter who was having her final exam in school, say—that she fails to notice the patient's need and neglects it. Under normal circumstances (say the nurse is not overworked, etc.), this is a case in which the nurse's neglect is neither justified nor excused but we may still have some understanding for the nurse's mistake, so that her worrying about her daughter counts as a mitigating consideration—as opposed to, say, a nurse who can't be bothered getting up because the football has just started. The latter also has *a* reason, but not one that we should consider as mitigating her failure of care.

Once we understand these distinctions properly, we also see that it is not that important to establish in which of these cases we can properly talk of responsibility: still, it seems clear that mitigation does not exclude responsibility; for both justification and excuse we may either speak of blameless responsibility or of lack of responsibility (that's a philosophical intricacy which we do not need to resolve here). What's more important is the following consideration: all three (justification, excuse, and mitigation) are normative terms, which goes to show that whether or not someone is responsible is a normative issue and not just an issue of whether or not someone acted. As we anticipated, there are cases in which we act but still we are not responsible, as many of the examples above show.

Are there also cases in which we are responsible for something which is not an action of ours? To answer this question, we should first look at cases which are, possibly, in between: namely the cases of ignorance and negligence (recklessness). Those are cases in which our actions bring about something that we did not intend to bring about. A particularly nasty case of ignorance—within healthcare—is so-called *never events*, clinical mistakes that should have never have happened (see chapter 5 for more details on never events and also some statistics about the occurrence).

CASE STUDY III: The Wrong Kidney

Imagine a surgeon who successfully removes the wrong kidney, for example. We can suppose that she has been misinformed: still, she acted intentionally. In Davidson's terms, she intentionally removed the kidney but unintentionally removed the left kidney (as she was supposed to remove the right one, we will suppose). Her ignorance of either the fact that she was actually supposed to remove the right one or of the fact that she was operating on the left one (less likely, we will admit) explains her mistake; other circumstances will determine, as we have seen above, whether she should be held responsible for her mistake—ignorance alone does not necessarily mean that the agent is or isn't responsible; it crucially depends on the circumstances of her ignorance.

One such crucial circumstance is whether her ignorance is negligent or culpable. Simplifying, if she was given false or inaccurate information by one of her colleagues and she could not have reasonably been expected to realize the inaccuracy of it or double check it, then her ignorance is not negligent or culpable; if, on the other hand, she was too busy with her own plans for the weekend while being briefed so that she missed some crucial information, then that's no justification or excuse and given the gravity of her mistake her absent-mindedness cannot be considered a mitigating consideration either, so that she is both fully responsible and liable for the relevant punishment. Still, we would not say that she acted intentionally: the more appropriate description of her behaviour is that she unintentionally operated on the left (and wrong) kidney but the circumstances of her unintentional action would be—in the latter case—such that she is fully responsible while—in the former case—we would excuse her and rather blame the colleague who provided inaccurate information.

There is an important consequence to this that should be emphasized: having acted unintentionally does not necessarily bear on the issue of responsibility as it does not necessarily constitute a justification, excuse or mitigating consideration.

What we have said so far should have also made it clear that an event does not need to be an action in order for someone to be responsible for that event. We can be made responsible for events that we did not prevent if it was reasonable to expect from us that we would or should have prevented it. These kinds of cases are particularly interesting because they highlight an important feature of responsibility, namely that more than one person can be responsible for something. So that if we did not prevent an event that we should have prevented, both the person who caused or otherwise brought about the event and also we ourselves having failed to prevent the event are responsible for what happened (whether the originator—so to speak—is more responsible than we are is a different issue).

Go back to our nurse scenario: suppose you are also a nurse who happens to go past that particular ward while your colleague is busy watching football and neglecting a needy patient. If you notice the needy patient but ignore it as well on the grounds that it is your colleague's responsibility rather than yours, it is reasonable to suppose that at least under certain circumstances (say you are not rushing to some other emergency) you make yourself thereby complicit in the neglect so that you are also responsible. You could have easily stopped or avoided the neglect, so that even though it was not your neglect to begin with, it becomes your neglect. But that, obviously, does not excuse your colleague who is watching football: simply, you are now both responsible for the neglect.

This scenario has another theoretical benefit: it shows that you can be made responsible for events that are not your actions, so that all that the original nurse does is watching football but given that watching football results in or causes the patient being neglected, the nurse is responsible for whatever happens to the patient as a result of her neglect even though she did not actually do those things. And clearly these cases also show that you can be responsible for omissions (whether or not omissions should be considered actions is again another matter here; on this question, see, e.g., Randolph Clarke's book *Omissions*[4]): for example, both nurses in the above case are responsible, we are supposing, for omitting to provide the relevant care.

We have learned a lot in this section: we have learned that you don't need to act intentionally in order to be held responsible (see negligence and ignorance); we have learned under what conditions you are not responsible (justification, excuse) or anyway blameless; and we have learned that there are cases in which you are responsible but may be spared punishment through mitigation. Finally, we have learned that more than one person can be responsible for the same event and that this kind of collective responsibility does not necessarily reduce the responsibility of each responsible agent.

Importantly, what we have learned also shows that mistakes or errors are neither necessarily excused nor necessarily negligent: the circumstances of these mistakes or errors will be crucial to whether or not we will be held responsible for them. One such circumstance is the answer to the following question: What did we know and what could have we been (reasonably) expected to know or find out? But those epistemic mistakes due to ignorance (which covers both false and incomplete/missing information) are not the only kind of mistake.

We may, for example, make a mistake because we are overworked or under pressure: again, depending on the precise circumstances, the fact that we are overworked or under pressure may count either as an excuse or as a mitigating factor. The theoretical character of this analysis makes it inevitable that we simplify a lot of the real-world problems related to responsibility and also responsibility attributions. But there are at least two elements that are particularly complicated and that should be flashed out: uncertainty and risk.

Healthcare professionals often have to deal with uncertainty: about diagnosis, about the effects of medication, and so on. It would be unfair to always speak of a mistake whenever something other than the event that healthcare professionals were hoping for or aiming at is realized. A mistake, then, is not just an unwanted consequence: it is an unwanted consequence whose occurrence could have been reasonably predicted or avoided—and the standard of reasonability will vary greatly here.

One final consideration about responsibility attribution which is particularly relevant to healthcare is that we don't want healthcare professionals to take any unwarranted risks with their patients' health but we also don't want healthcare professionals to be too careful in their clinical decision making just to avoid mistakes and thereby liability. The most beneficial healthcare environment for patients is one where practitioners are allowed to take reasonable risks in order to achieve the best possible healthcare outcome.

So while a focus on responsibility is both beneficial and inevitable, there is a limit to such focus that is hard to delineate precisely: an environment where playing it safe to avoid liability results in less than the healthcare provision which could have been expected. This is not a philosophical issue but rather a legal and political one so that I will not discuss it in any detail; but it was important to flag its relationship to the attribution of responsibility, because it shows that there is at least one important respect in which responsibility and its attributions are not ethically neutral but can rather interfere with successful healthcare provision.

Special Responsibility and the Hippocratic Oath

Do healthcare professionals have a special responsibility due to their knowledge and skills? For reasons that will become clear, I am going to start this section by introducing something that has been conspicuously missing from an ethics book for healthcare students and professionals: the Hippocratic Oath.

Figure 8.1 shows a recent translation of the Hippocratic Oath from the *National Library of Medicine* (from which we have also taken the Greek/Latin version above):

I swear by Apollo the physician, and Asclepius, and Hygieia and Panacea and all the gods and goddesses as my witnesses, that, according to my ability and judgement, I will keep this Oath and this contract:

To hold him who taught me this art equally dear to me as my parents, to be a partner in life with him, and to fulfill his needs when required; to look upon his offspring as equals to my own siblings, and to teach them this art, if they shall wish to learn it, without fee or contract; and that by the set rules, lectures, and every other mode of instruction, I will impart a knowledge of the art to my own sons, and those of my teachers, and to students bound by this contract and having sworn this Oath to the law of medicine, but to no others.

I will use those dietary regimens which will benefit my patients according to my greatest ability and judgement, and I will do no harm or injustice to them.

I will not give a lethal drug to anyone if I am asked, nor will I advise such a plan; and similarly I will not give a woman a pessary to cause an abortion.

In purity and according to divine law will I carry out my life and my art.

I will not use the knife, even upon those suffering from stones, but I will leave this to those who are trained in this craft.

Into whatever homes I go, I will enter them for the benefit of the sick, avoiding any voluntary act of impropriety or corruption, including the seduction of women or men, whether they are free men or slaves.

Whatever I see or hear in the lives of my patients, whether in connection with my professional practice or not, which ought not to be spoken of outside, I will keep secret, as considering all such things to be private.

So long as I maintain this Oath faithfully and without corruption, may it be granted to me to partake of life fully and the practice of my art, gaining the respect of all men for all time. However, should I transgress this Oath and violate it, may the opposite be my fate.[5]

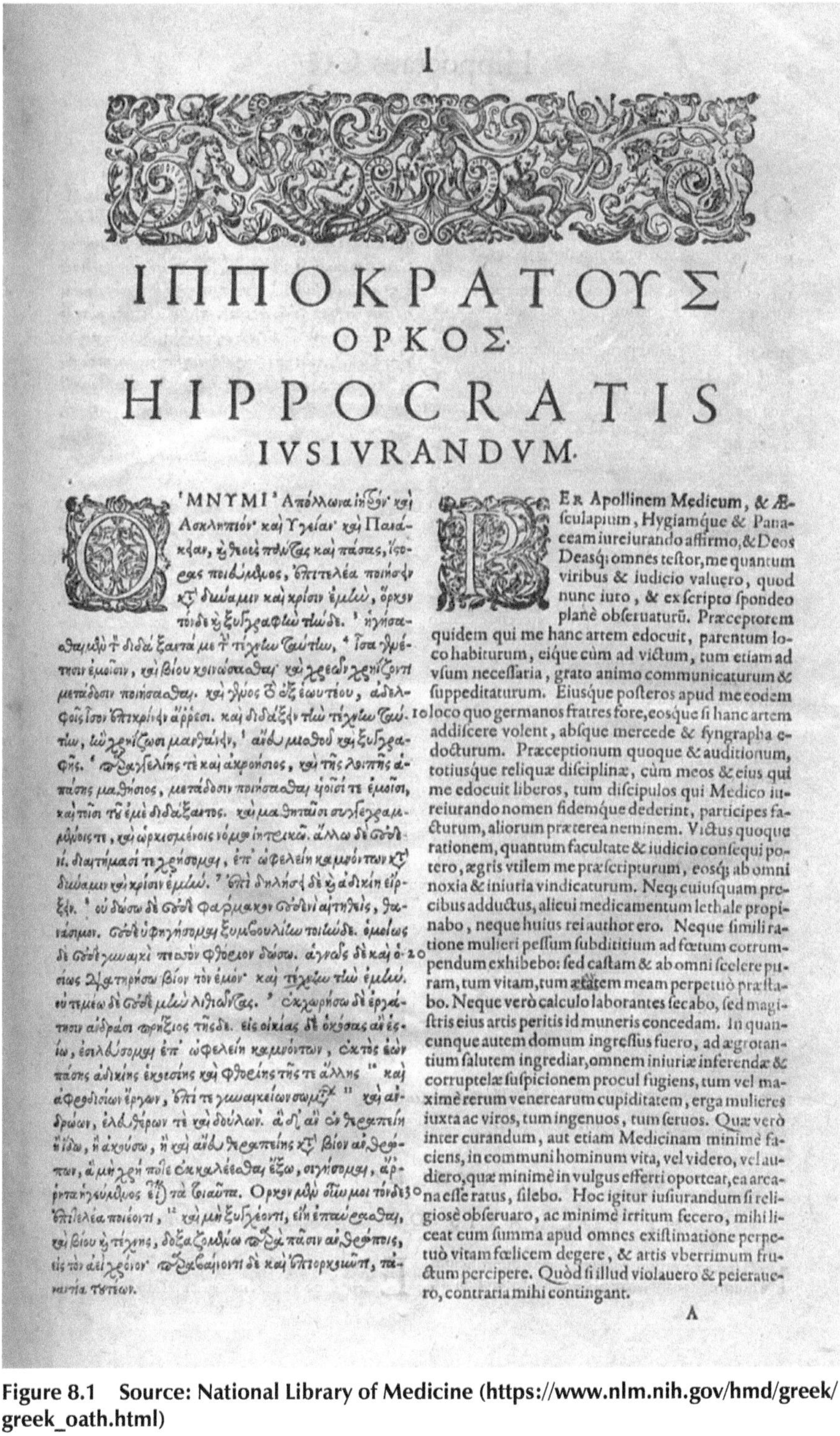
1

ΙΠΠΟΚΡΑΤΟΥΣ

ΟΡΚΟΣ.

HIPPOCRATIS

IVSIVRANDVM.

ΟΜΝΥΜΙ Ἀπόλλωνα ἰητρὸν καὶ Ἀσκληπιὸν καὶ Ὑγείαν καὶ Πανάκειαν, καὶ θεοὺς πάντας καὶ πάσας, ἵστορας ποιεύμενος, ἐπιτελέα ποιήσειν κατὰ δύναμιν καὶ κρίσιν ἐμὴν, ὅρκον τόνδε καὶ ξυγγραφὴν τήνδε. ἡγήσασθαι μὲν τὸν διδάξαντά με τὴν τέχνην ταύτην, ἴσα γενέτῃσιν ἐμοῖσιν, καὶ βίου κοινώσασθαι, καὶ χρεῶν χρηίζοντι μετάδοσιν ποιήσασθαι, καὶ γένος τὸ ἐξ ἑωυτοῦ, ἀδελφοῖς ἴσον ἐπικρινέειν ἄρρεσι, καὶ διδάξειν τὴν τέχνην ταύτην, ἢν χρηίζωσι μανθάνειν, ἄνευ μισθοῦ καὶ ξυγγραφῆς. παραγγελίης τε καὶ ἀκροήσιος, καὶ τῆς λοιπῆς ἁπάσης μαθήσιος, μετάδοσιν ποιήσασθαι υἱοῖσί τε ἐμοῖσι, καὶ τοῖσι τοῦ ἐμὲ διδάξαντος, καὶ μαθηταῖσι συγγεγραμμένοισί τε, καὶ ὡρκισμένοις νόμῳ ἰητρικῷ. ἄλλῳ δὲ οὐδενί. διαιτήμασί τε χρήσομαι, ἐπ' ὠφελείῃ καμνόντων κατὰ δύναμιν καὶ κρίσιν ἐμήν. ἐπὶ δηλήσει δὲ καὶ ἀδικίῃ εἴρξειν. οὐ δώσω δὲ οὐδὲ φάρμακον οὐδενὶ αἰτηθεὶς, θανάσιμον. οὐδὲ ὑφηγήσομαι ξυμβουλίην τοιήνδε. ὁμοίως δὲ οὐδὲ γυναικὶ πεσσὸν φθόριον δώσω. ἁγνῶς δὲ καὶ ὁσίως διατηρήσω βίον τὸν ἐμὸν καὶ τέχνην τὴν ἐμήν. οὐ τεμέω δὲ οὐδὲ μὴν λιθιῶντας. ἐκχωρήσω δὲ ἐργάτῃσιν ἀνδράσι πρήξιος τῆσδε. εἰς οἰκίας δὲ ὁκόσας ἂν ἐσίω, ἐσελεύσομαι ἐπ' ὠφελείῃ καμνόντων, ἐκτὸς ἐὼν πάσης ἀδικίης ἑκουσίης καὶ φθορίης τῆς τε ἄλλης καὶ ἀφροδισίων ἔργων, ἐπί τε γυναικείων σωμάτων καὶ ἀνδρώων, ἐλευθέρων τε καὶ δούλων. ἃ δ' ἂν ἐν θεραπείῃ ἴδω, ἢ ἀκούσω, ἢ καὶ ἄνευ θεραπείης κατὰ βίον ἀνθρώπων, ἃ μὴ χρή ποτε ἐκλαλέεσθαι ἔξω, σιγήσομαι, ἄρρητα ἡγεύμενος εἶναι τὰ τοιαῦτα. Ὅρκον μὲν οὖν μοι τόνδε ἐπιτελέα ποιέοντι, καὶ μὴ ξυγχέοντι, εἴη ἐπαύρασθαι, καὶ βίου καὶ τέχνης, δοξαζομένῳ παρὰ πᾶσιν ἀνθρώποις, ἐς τὸν αἰεὶ χρόνον· παραβαίνοντι δὲ καὶ ἐπιορκοῦντι, τἀναντία τούτων.

PER Apollinem Medicum, & Æsculapium, Hygiamque & Panaceam iureiurando affirmo, & Deos Deasq; omnes testor, me quantum viribus & iudicio valuero, quod nunc iuro, & ex scripto spondeo planè obseruaturū. Præceptorem quidem qui me hanc artem edocuit, parentum loco habiturum, eique cùm ad victum, tum etiam ad vsum necessaria, grato animo communicaturum & suppeditaturum. Eiusque posteros apud me eodem loco quo germanos fratres fore, eosque si hanc artem addiscere volent, absque mercede & syngrapha edocturum. Præceptionum quoque & auditionum, totiusque reliquæ disciplinæ, cùm meos & eius qui me edocuit liberos, tum discipulos qui Medico iureiurando nomen fidemque dederint, participes facturum, aliorum præterea neminem. Victus quoque rationem, quantum facultate & iudicio consequi potero, ægris vtilem me præscripturum, eosq; ab omni noxia & iniuria vindicaturum. Neq; cuiusquam precibus adductus, alicui medicamentum lethale propinabo, neque huius rei author ero. Neque simili ratione mulieri pessum subdititium ad fœtum corrumpendum exhibebo: sed castam & ab omni scelere puram, tum vitam, tum artem meam perpetuò præstabo. Neque verò calculo laborantes secabo, sed magistris eius artis peritis id muneris concedam. In quancunque autem domum ingressus fuero, ad ægrotantium salutem ingrediar, omnem iniuriæ inferendæ & corruptelæ suspicionem procul fugiens, tum vel maximè rerum venerearum cupiditatem, erga mulieres iuxta ac viros, tum ingenuos, tum seruos. Quæ verò inter curandum, aut etiam Medicinam minimè faciens, in communi hominum vita, vel videro, vel audiero, quæ minimè in vulgus efferri oporteat, ea arcana esse ratus, silebo. Hoc igitur iusiurandum si religiosè obseruaro, ac minimè irritum fecero, mihi liceat cum summa apud omnes existimatione perpetuò vitam fœlicem degere, & artis vberrimum fructum percipere. Quòd si illud violauero & peierauero, contraria mihi contingant.

A

Figure 8.1 Source: National Library of Medicine (https://www.nlm.nih.gov/hmd/greek/greek_oath.html)

A modern version of the oath was (re)written in 1964 by Louis Lasagna, academic dean of the School of Medicine at Tufts University (this version is used in many medical schools today):

I swear to fulfill, to the best of my ability and judgment, this covenant:

I will respect the hard-won scientific gains of those physicians in whose steps I walk, and gladly share such knowledge as is mine with those who are to follow.

I will apply, for the benefit of the sick, all measures [that] are required, avoiding those twin traps of overtreatment and therapeutic nihilism.

I will remember that there is art to medicine as well as science, and that warmth, sympathy, and understanding may outweigh the surgeon's knife or the chemist's drug.

I will not be ashamed to say "I know not," nor will I fail to call in my colleagues when the skills of another are needed for a patient's recovery.

I will respect the privacy of my patients, for their problems are not disclosed to me that the world may know. Most especially must I tread with care in matters of life and death. If it is given me to save a life, all thanks. But it may also be within my power to take a life; this awesome responsibility must be faced with great humbleness and awareness of my own frailty. Above all, I must not play at God.

I will remember that I do not treat a fever chart, a cancerous growth, but a sick human being, whose illness may affect the person's family and economic stability. My responsibility includes these related problems, if I am to care adequately for the sick.

I will prevent disease whenever I can, for prevention is preferable to cure.

I will remember that I remain a member of society, with special obligations to all my fellow human beings, those sound of mind and body as well as the infirm.

If I do not violate this oath, may I enjoy life and art, respected while I live and remembered with affection thereafter. May I always act so as to preserve the finest traditions of my calling and may I long experience the joy of healing those who seek my help.

The reason why I am including the Hippocratic Oath is, I must confess, not its content, which I take to be, at least from a philosophical point of view, no more than a fun curiosity. Rather, I think that the lasting existence (the oath is thought to be from the late fifth century BC) and continuous influence of the oath are symbolic of the hypothesis that we shall investigate in this section, namely the idea that healthcare professionals have some sort of special responsibility (to care, for example); what is often referred to as the *duty of care*.

At a time when there were yet no written contracts, physicians were already expected to take an oath—this alone suggests that from antiquity onwards, members of the medical profession were held to higher—or at least different—standards than other professionals. The question before us in this section is not the historical one about the accuracy of this hypothesis but the philosophical one of whether this hypothesis, whatever its history, has any theoretical plausibility.

CASE STUDY IV: 'Is There a Doctor on Board?'

To begin with, let us distinguish between different possible senses of special responsibility. Take the infamous 'is there a doctor on board?': on the one hand, special responsibility may just mean that, if you are the only one around with certain skills, you have a responsibility to make these skills available. So if you are the only doctor on board you have a responsibility to help; the same would apply to the case in which you are the only midwife in case a woman is about to deliver her baby or, say, if you are the only one with a pilot's license in a case in which both pilots have suddenly been incapacitated or died. It is quickly clear that, if this is the sense in which healthcare professionals have special responsibilities, then those responsibilities are not really special, everyone may have this responsibility in particular circumstances given their own skills' set (well, it is admittedly more difficult to generate a case in which a philosopher like myself may have those kinds of special responsibilities, though).

Alternatively, we may think of special responsibility in the sense of being obliged to do more than others, given one's talents. The idea would be the following: if you are trying to decide whether to undertake an acting career or a medical career, it may be plausible to add the following caveat to your career plans. If you opt for a medical career, the resulting talents will not be such that you can every time decide, according to your inclination, whether or not to deploy those talents. The same will not apply to an acting career: the resulting talents do not oblige you to anything in particular, you will always be able to decide whether or not to use them and for what purpose.

We now see that this question of the special responsibility of healthcare professionals, obscure as it is, is basically the question of whether the healthcare profession is just any other profession or whether it comes with some particular strings attached—ethical strings, in this case (and this in turn explains why I have started this section with the Hippocratic Oath).

The point is not even that controversial when you think of it: if you train as a doctor, it just happens to be the case that the life-saving skills that you acquire will be such that, sometimes, you will not be allowed to refuse to use them; and that's just because those skills are, indeed, life-saving. We can be very liberal and concede that acting skills and medical skills should be considered equal and still it will be, empirically speaking, not very often that one's acting skills will be in a position to save lives while that will probably happen to just about every doctor during a lifetime—whether on duty or not. And this is, by the way, another way of characterizing the special responsibility of healthcare professionals: that they have a duty to make their skills available—given some medical emergency—independently of whether they are on or off duty.

Again, this does not have to be conceived as some special priority status for the medical profession: it could just be taken to be an empirical fact that medical skills will be required more often and more urgently than acting skills or, for that matter, financial skills.

This kind of special responsibility can lead to all sorts of problems: once you get involved in an emergency, whether on duty or off duty, you may make yourself liable if you make a mistake; and explaining that you weren't on duty at the time and got involved voluntarily will not necessarily get you off the hook, either morally or even legally.

I was personally present when the following happened: a large group of people had gathered in the mountains to listen to a string concert, the nearest road being at least half an hour mountain-path away. Soon after the concert had started, an elderly man who had walked up the mountain suffered a heart attack; people—including at least one doctor—tried to help. My understanding is that a helicopter was alerted and then called off because the doctor did not think the patient could be saved. Much later an ambulance managed to make its way up the mountain path—the patient was still alive when the ambulance took him off but died later that day in hospital.

Here the question is not whether the doctor present at the scene made a mistake in calling off the helicopter—he probably did but I am not in a position to tell and, as far as I know, an inquiry is underway. The more basic ethical point here is that the doctor got involved and, indeed, according to what we have said in this section may have even had a responsibility (at least morally speaking) to get involved and to try to help given a special duty of care; but once he got involved, then he became responsible for subsequent decisions—and importantly this is true whether or not he had a responsibility to begin with. So that we have a dilemma, in which a doctor may be better off not getting involved in the first place.

Here is another standard case to illustrate the above point, taken from US legal practice:

CASE STUDY V: *A Doctor Dining in a Restaurant*

A physician must owe a duty of care to patients before his or her competency in performing that duty can be judged. In US jurisprudence, a person has no affirmative duty to assist injured individuals in the absence of a special relationship with them (such as doctor–patient, attorney–client, guardian–ward, etc.). A doctor dining in a restaurant has no duty to come forward and assist a fellow customer who is suffering a heart attack. If the doctor merely continues with his meal and does nothing to help, the ailing person would not have an action for malpractice against him, not-withstanding their harm. However, once a doctor voluntarily decides to assist others or come to their aid, he or she becomes liable for any injury that results from any negligence during that assistance.[6]

A couple of distinctions are in order here: first of all, we should distinguish between the question of whether an off-duty doctor has a moral responsibility to intervene and the question of whether an off-duty doctor has a legal responsibility to intervene; the above suggests that at least in the United States, off-duty doctors have, at best, a moral responsibility to intervene but that, as far as the law is concerned, they are allowed to stay put and continue their dinner. The second point is what follows from a moral or legal responsibility to intervene: we have seen that in US legal practice even though there is no legal responsibility to intervene, if the off-duty doctor voluntarily decides to get involved, he or she will be legally liable for any resulting mistakes—as calling off the helicopter in the case I have presented.

An interesting question is the following: given that there is no legal obligation to intervene for an off-duty doctor, does the fact that that doctor is liable for any resulting mistake depend on some implicit or explicit moral or ethical obligation (or at least expectation) that he or she intervene? After all, compare the medical case with the following nonmedical case: you ask a friend to help you relocate; your friend agrees to help and, while he is helping you relocate, he drops an expensive lamp. It seems as though it would be at the very least unfair, from a moral point of view, to expect compensation from your friend—even though insurance companies may think otherwise. Why should we think differently in the medical case? Two options here: on the one hand, that we think differently in the medical case may indeed suggest that the medical professional has some priority, resulting in this case in a moral duty to get involved for an off-duty doctor; alternatively, we may think that there is no difference between the medical case and the relocation case, so that in both cases there is no moral obligation to compensate; both parties got involved voluntarily and it would therefore be unfair to blame them.

Whichever of the above two options we take, we should note at least two final elements: a doctor's special responsibility or duty of care is subject to the same worry that we had in the previous section, namely that responsibility attributions are not ethically neutral but may rather disincentivize action and even moderate risk taking—we want doctors in these emergency situations to get involved, not to keep silent and pretend they are philosophers. The second point is that the supposed duty of care that comes with particular healthcare skills is a burden but one that is, crucially, freely chosen along with medical training and the medical profession. Whether or not it is a burden worth carrying, that is your decision alone.

Summary

In this final chapter, we have analysed the crucial ethical concept of responsibility and applied it to healthcare. We have distinguished between intentional actions and mistakes while showing that one can be responsible whether or not one has acted intentionally, and that whether someone is responsible for his or her mistake will depend on normative considerations such as recklessness. Also, we have borrowed some important concepts from the philosophy of law to further distinguish between different possibilities within healthcare: specifically, Hart's tripartite distinction between justification, excuses, and mitigating considerations. The chapter concludes with a discussion of whether healthcare professionals have a special responsibility of care.

Notes

1. See Donald Davidson, *Essays on Actions and Events* (Oxford: Oxford University Press, 1980).

2. H. L. A. Hart, *Punishment and Responsibility: Essays in the Philosophy of Law* (Oxford: Oxford University Press, 1968).

3. Ibid., 13–14.

4. Randolph Clarke, *Omissions* (Oxford: Oxford University Press, 2014).

5. Translated by Michael North, National Library of Medicine, 2002: https://www.nlm.nih.gov/hmd/greek/greek_oath.html. The picture is also taken from the *National Library of Medicine* website above.

6. http://www.findlaw.com/.

Bibliography

Aas, Sean (2016). 'Disabled—Therefore, Unhealthy?' *Ethical Theory and Moral Practice* 19 (5): 1259–74.

Beauchamp, T. L. and J. F. Childress (2012). *Principles of Biomedical Ethics*. Seventh edition. Oxford University Press.

Clarke, R. (2014). *Omissions*. Oxford: Oxford University Press.

Crigger, B. J. (1998). *Cases in Bioethics*. New York: Macmillan.

Dancy, J. (1983). 'Ethical Particularism and Morally Relevant Properties', *Mind* 92:530–47.

———. (1993). *Moral Reasons*. Oxford: Blackwell.

———. (2004). *Ethics without Principles*. Oxford: Clarendon Press.

Davidson, D. (1980). *Essays on Actions and Events*. Oxford: Oxford University Press.

Di Nucci, E. (2014). 'Addiction, Compulsion, and Agency'. *Neuroethics* 7 (1): 105–07.

———. (2014). *Ethics Without Intention*. London: Bloomsbury.

Fabre, C. (2006). *Whose Body Is It Anyway?* Oxford: Oxford University Press.

Grill, K., and K. Voigt (2016). 'The Case for Banning Cigarettes'. *Journal of Medical Ethics* 42:293–301.

Hart, H. L. A. (1968). *Punishment and Responsibility: Essays in the Philosophy of Law*. Oxford: Oxford University Press.

Kant, I. (1785/1996). *Groundwork of the Metaphysics of Morals*. Translated by M. Gregor. Cambridge: Cambridge University Press.

Keller, S. (2013). *Partiality*. Princeton, NJ: Princeton University Press.

Leiter, B. (2012). *Why Tolerate Religion?* Princeton, NJ: Princeton University Press.

Lippert-Rasmussen, K. (2016). *Luck Egalitarianism*. London: Bloomsbury.

Marquis, D. (1989). 'Why Abortion is Immoral'. *The Journal of Philosophy* 86 (4): 183–202.

McEwan, I. (2014). *The Children Act*. London: Jonathan Cape.

Mill, J. S. (1863). *Utilitarianism*. London: Parker, Son, and Bourn.

Miller, F., and A. Wertheimer, eds. (2010). *The Ethics of Consent: Theory and Practice*. Oxford: Oxford University Press.

Pickard, H. (2012). 'The Purpose in Chronic Addiction'. *AJOB Neuroscience* 3 (2): 40–49.

Quine, W. V. O. (1951). 'Two Dogmas of Empiricism'. *The Philosophical Review* 60 (1): 20–43.

Rawls, J. (1971). *A Theory of Justice*. Cambridge, MA: Harvard University Press.

Segall, S (2009). *Health, Luck, and Justice*. Princeton, NJ: Princeton University Press.

Singer, P. (1972). 'Famine Affluence and Morality', *Philosophy and Public Affairs* 1, no. 3 (Spring, 1972): 229–43.

Strawson, P. F. (2008). *Freedom and Resentment and Other Essays*. London: Routledge.

Thomson, J. J. (1971). 'A Defense of Abortion'. *Philosophy and Public Affairs* 1 (1): 47–66.

———. (1985). 'The Trolley Problem'. *The Yale Law Journal* 94 (6): 1395.

Tredennick, H., and H. Tredennick, trans. (1954/1993). *The Last Days of Socrates*. London: Penguin.

Velleman, D. (2015). *Beyond Price: Essays on Birth and Death*. Cambridge: OpenBook Publishers.

Williams, B. (1972). *Morality*. Cambridge: Cambridge University Press.

Index

www.ingramcontent.com/pod-product-compliance
Ingram Content Group UK Ltd.
Pitfield, Milton Keynes, MK11 3LW, UK
UKHW012041150926
475560UK00001B/119

9 781786 608697